50 & FIT

Build muscle. Burn fat.
Eat right. Repeat...

50 & FIT

Build muscle. Burn fat. Eat right. Repeat...

BY JACK REDMOND, M.Ed.

Redmond Strategy Group

www.RedmondStrategyGroup.com

Lose Weight and Increase Daily Energy Levels

DISCLAIMER: This book contains advice on exercise, nutrition and stress management. It is recommended that anyone seeking to make health changes including exercise, nutrition and stress management seek a physician's approval and advice. Principles and methods of weight loss, nutritional habits and stress management etc. are not meant to replace medical or therapeutic care. All efforts have been made to ensure all information contained within this book is accurate. Both author and Redmond Strategy Group disclaim liability for any medical outcomes that may occur as a result of applying principles and methods described or suggested in this book.

50 & FIT
Build muscle. Burn fat. Eat right. Repeat...

Copyright © 2020—Jack Redmond

www.RedmondStrategyGroup.com

Cover and interior layout: swinghouse design studios

Cover photo credits: ©iStockphoto [south_agency, filadendron, svariophoto]

isbn: 9798668867868

printed in the United States of America

ACKNOWLEDGMENT

So much goes into a book! In some ways, this book is a history lane of my life. Here are a few key people who have journeyed with me along the way where I learned how the body responds to exercise by both doing and studying.

Donovan Brown – my high school linebacker coach who picked me up at 5:45 am before school to lift weights and taught me how to push harder to build muscle! You taught me to dig deeper every day in practice and don't forget those occasional "cooker" sessions!

MY TRAINING PARTNERS

HIGH SCHOOL

Alex Pedre – he was the strongest guy I could find, so I trained with him. He taught me the value of having a training partner who was stronger than you and the value of people pushing each other to be better.

COLLEGE

Mario Gallucio – we ate and trained and ate and trained. One summer we literally trained 2-3 times a day for 40 minutes and ate 6-8 times a day. Overtraining was simply undereating on the Bulgarian Powerburst training system! We trained at Gold's Gym in Toms River, NJ.

Aron Basile – my college lifting partner and roommate for four years. How did you ever put up with me? We trained at Powerhouse in Deptford, NJ.

MY EDUCATION

Chuck Whedon A.T.C., – Rowan University, Athletic Training 1988-1993 – you taught me how the body worked, adapted and healed.

Dr. DeMeersman, Teachers College, Columbia University – thank you for teaching how the body adapts on a cellular and muscular level to nutrition and exercise.

MY WEIGHT LOSS COACHES

Bristol Jenkins and E.J. Frain – for the phone conversations, talking through, and teaching me about intermittent fasting, Keto and encouraging me when things got tough. Also, for the tough love, pushing me through my fragile ego, and for teaching an old dog a few new tricks!

MY EDITING TEAM

Amanda Rooker for coaching me on the final transcript, **Jennifer Hanchey** for line editing and **Angie Kiesling** for the final proofread.

MY GRAPHIC DESIGNER

George Rodriguez and the crew over at swinghouse design studio (swinghousedesign.com) for the creation and design of the book cover and all internal formatting. Thanks for making me and the book look good!

MY CHIROPRACTIC AND PT TEAM

Thank you **Dr. Alfred Davis Jr., Chiropractor Clinical Director, Dr. Akwete Sackey, Chiropractor Associate and Peter Kofitsas, MS, PT from Davis Integrated Medicine** in Montclair, NJ. Looking back, I'm not sure how I lost the final 20 pounds or so with a sprained spine! With Peter's PT and Dr. Sackey ongoing treatment and Dr. Davis jumping in at key moments, your team made it possible!

ACKNOWLEDGMENT

ENDORSEMENTS

In his book *50 & Fit*, author Jack Redmond takes a simple and effective approach to regaining your health and returning to your ideal weight. His strategies are clear and effective regardless of how much you want to lose and any obstacles you may be facing. It is full of valuable information that will meet you where you are at and take you on a journey to fitness and good health!

His book is inspirational and full of information that people can immediately apply. I am so happy that our facility played a role in helping to heal injuries and correct subluxations in his journey to get well and hit his weight loss goal.

Dr. Alfred Davis Jr., D.C., DACBSP, DAAPM, FICC, CME
Director, Davis Integrated Medicine, Montclair, NJ
www.DavisIntegratedMedicine.com

In *50 & Fit*, Jack Redmond helps you paint a picture of a better life where you can be thinner, fitter and have more energy each and every day. But he doesn't stop there. He gives simple step by step processes based on scientific principle and practical experience. *50 & Fit* can help anyone look and feel better!

> **Bristol Jenkins, CSCS, AFAA, FMS**
> Nutrition Certified – The National Association of Certified
>   Natural Health Professionals
> Bodies by Bristol: Owner and Operator
> www.BodiesbyBristol.com

Jack Redmond teaches people real life strategies essential to get fit and be healthy. Jack shares the principles and process he personally used to lose 40 pounds. *50 & Fit* can coach you by keeping it simple and applicable by first helping you believe that your fitness goals are possible, then guiding you to achieve your goals by following simple and practical principles.

> **Lighting Speed Athletics – Owner and Operator**
> ACE Certified Personal Trainer, Speed Coach
> Contact by Social Media *@LightningSpeedAthletics*

I have known Jack since my first day of school, yep, kindergarten. He is super smart, down to earth, has an exceptional work ethic, and a man of great character. We trained together for football throughout high school. I literally watched him build his body as a teenager with the very principles he utilized to lose 40 lbs. and build muscle over three decades later! As a health practitioner and advocate, I highly recommend Jack Redmond's *50 & Fit* to anyone interested in improving their fitness and getting healthier.

Scott J Lloyd, DC, CMT, CCWP
Cafe of Life Chiropractic – Owner/Operator
Brick, NJ
www.ScottLloyd.info

Jack helped me make tremendous progress on my weight loss leading up to my 50th birthday. His simple and practical advice helped shift my body to a fat burning machine. I have more energy and simply feel better. He told me I could do it and I believe his practical expertise can lead to that weight loss you have wanted for a long time.

Malik Carey, CEO, Founder
www.FamilyHealingCenterNJ.com

ENDORSEMENTS

FOREWORD

Hitting the nail on the head is no easy detail. To do so with the epidemic of weight gain, which so many struggle with, and to do so with passion and accuracy is not commonplace. Jack Redmond has done so here, but to say I am surprised would be a lie.

However, at the beginning of my relationship with Jack in 1989, I would've been quite surprised to learn he would go on to write such an exceptional book. Let me explain why. I was part of a push to meet accreditation standards for the athletic training program at Glassboro State College, now Rowan University. As always, I was attempting to draw the most talented and impassioned students into a career that I still feel has the most potential of any health care profession to holistically impact patient health.

A number of bright students were in the program already, and perhaps three times more had withdrawn because of the rigor of study. In my haste, I first categorized Mr. Redmond in the latter group, and I do admit to a degree of academic profiling. You see, at that point in his life, to say it mildly, Jack was a little rough around the edges, still embracing the role of rebel. Despite his intensity and success on the football field, I could not see him fitting the mold of the health care practitioner. With long scraggly hair, cut-off T-shirts that displayed some serious guns, and a seemingly uncontainable enthusiasm toward both football and life, my estimate was that this young man, who looked like a Neanderthal, had bleak prospects of becoming an effective athletic trainer or role model for youth. My estimate was off.

Though very articulate, Jack had a barely contained energy that seemed a bit over the top for professional life. Yet my nature was to give kids the benefit of the doubt and let the academic rigor of the didactic classes and clinical education components weed out the weaker students. To my surprise, Jack raked in A after A on quizzes, tests, and projects, demonstrating an intellect quite suited for health care. I learned that what he initially lacked in professionalism, he made up with passion and excellence as a student and practitioner.

He quickly mastered and retained the basic concepts of anatomy pathology and was able to apply that information to the athletes we treated and returned to the school's nationally competitive sports program. His status as a standout football player and intense demeanor meant he related well to the student athletes—especially the hard-headed football players—who walked into our incredibly busy sports medicine clinic. It certainly did not hurt that he was literally "jacked" in appearance like a professional body builder, but it was his impassioned interaction with patients, coaches, and faculty alike that set him apart.

His professional dress was still lacking, though I was so impressed with his ability and potential that I let it go as the demand of my position dictated prioritizing. Several years later, when he stated his desire to get a master's degree at an Ivy League school and asked if I would help him forge that path, I made it clear that his unrefined appearance and bigger-than-life personality would need to be addressed. And addressed they were, instantly.

I introduced him to some Ivy League colleagues, and he did the rest, securing a graduate assistantship and continuing on to pursue his dream. Just imagine the pride I felt in having some part in this young man's discovery of a career passion, drive toward academic success, and personal transformation.

During the next twenty years of my career as a college professor, I would get snippets of Jack's progress, his practice in athletic training and ministry. I followed closely the blossoming I couldn't have fathomed when I first met Jack. However, none of this achievement is surprising at all now that I truly know this man.

Thus, I can enthusiastically endorse this manuscript. Jack touches on all the main points for making significant lifestyle changes and making them stick. The text demonstrates his mastery of human physiology and, more so, his understanding of the physical, psychological, and spiritual elements of life that must move in sync to produce sustainable, permanent results. I am by nature a skeptic and realize thousands of health-related self-help books have already been offered to the public. But very few have been authored by someone who not only has forged through the life-changing processes themselves but also has the academic background to lend legitimacy to the words.

Jack's plan is well thought-out and comprehensive yet flexible enough to apply to anyone looking for positive lifestyle change. Do yourself a favor: embody the passion and technical details of this well-planned tool to gain the success a small minority have the pleasure of experiencing.

Chuck Whedon, MS, LAT, ATC, CSCS
Coordinator of Clinical Education/Specialist Professor,
  Monmouth University
Prior: Associate AD Sports Medicine; 2012-2015
Sports Medicine Staff, Football and Swimming, 2015-2018

Coordinator of Athletic Training, Instructor in AT, Rowan University, 1986-2012; Retired

CONTENTS

INTRODUCTION

I started to hate how I felt each day. Some days I was exhausted by eight in the morning. I kept gaining weight, and my body hurt in new ways. I also sensed my body getting weaker. Things were headed in the wrong direction. Then it happened. My wife stopped arguing with me, and I knew I was in trouble. A couple of times over the past five to ten years, I had shared that I had gained another five pounds, and she would encourage me and say she didn't notice, that it was no big deal. When I explained I had gained thirty-five pounds since we got married, her eyes got big. She pressed her lips together and simply walked away.

As I closed in on fifty, my body was changing. Specifically, my daily energy was decreasing and my bodyweight increasing. And I'm not alone. Just about every man I know complains about weight gain and energy loss. Many knock on my door to seek help in losing weight, and this has nothing to do with my actual job. Many women also ask for guidance to lose weight and increase daily energy. It was crystal clear: I had knowledge I needed to implement in my life and also share with others.

I KNOW BETTER

One problem with this picture is that I am highly trained in physiology and nutrition, earning multiple master's degrees in applied physiology from Columbia University after an undergraduate degree in health and physical education with a specialization in athletic training from Rowan University. The painful reality was that my behavior did not match my knowledge. Throughout this book, we will consider how behavior is almost always more important than knowledge alone.

On November 19, 2018, I stepped on the scale and weighed 225 pounds. Overall, I was healthy and in better shape than many—if not most of—my peers, but honestly, I was overweight. I had slowly gained weight and felt like I was on a slippery slope. I graduated high school weighing 190 pounds and spent the next couple of years purposely gaining muscle to play college football, reaching 226 pounds After football, I purposely cut down to 190 pounds as I studied physiology and nutrition at Columbia University. I know more about being physically healthy than 99.9 percent of humans, but knowledge alone isn't enough. I felt embarrassed by my condition. I have the knowledge to help you, but this is also my personal journey. I am walking it out with you.

Most people I know would have said I was okay—you know, not too fat. I joked about fighting the "dad bod," but it wasn't funny anymore. I was losing the battle. The dad bod was slapping me around! My heaviest weight at age twenty-two was 226 pounds after being a college middle linebacker, force-feeding myself for ten years and lifting weights three to six times per week. Then at forty-eight, I weighed 226 pounds again, but let's just say, it wasn't the same 226 pounds. Roughly twenty-five years later, I had transformed from a physical specimen to the guy who wouldn't take his shirt off in public.

In many ways, my story is "our" story. Male or female, we fight this common battle. The details are unique, but we have traveled the same general path. Time and life's circumstances result in slow and steady unwanted weight gain. On top of that, as you age, energy levels tend to decrease, especially if you are carrying around unnecessary weight.

Though I will never impress people with my physique as I did a few decades back, I want to be healthy and in control of my weight—instead of letting my weight control me. It's ironic because I spent so much of my youth trying to gain weight; now, it just happens. It's reality. It's life, but I refuse to accept it.

I am surrounded by men and women on the same journey. The vast majority of people I talk to want more daily energy and to lose at least fifteen to twenty pounds. We are not trying to be models; we just want to live well.

At forty-eight, I made a decision to lose thirty-five pounds. I committed to go from 225 to 190 pounds, writing about my experience along the way. Ironically, when I committed to this, I immediately gained three pounds. I had to laugh, but then I got serious.

If, like me, you are tired of passively gaining weight while suffering from less energy, negative emotions, physical pain, and even deteriorating health, then it's time to make changes. Losing weight is simple—not easy but simple. With weight loss, improved diet, and better conditioning, you can also have more energy each and every day as you drop unwanted weight.

OUR THREE-STEP GAME PLAN

I want to help you win. To win, you need a winning game plan. It should be clear, simple, and effective. Here is our three-step plan:

1. **Build muscle:** Muscle is your fat-burning engine.

2. **Burn fat:** Through specific exercise and food choices, we'll target fat.

3. **Eat right:** You'll learn to make good choices and eat at optimal times.

If you consistently and deliberately do these three things, you can reach your goal. My confidence is based on scientific and physiological principles you can depend on. These principles will get results now and help you stay at your goal weight when finished.

50 & Fit captures my journey from 228 pounds to 188 pounds. Though your journey may be smaller or larger, you can run your race and win.

You can make lasting changes, lose unwanted fat, and feel better. The goal is not perfection but to be the best you can be. I am just an average guy fighting a common fight, but I've made the changes, and I am here to coach you.

As a life coach and president and founder of Redmond Strategy

Group (www.RedmondStrategyGroup.com), I follow a simple three-step process to pursue and achieve any goal. I will consistently refer back to these steps: dream, plan, and execute. Let's apply these steps to our weight-loss goal:

1. **Dream:** Having a vivid picture and vision will motivate you to success.

2. **Plan:** Understanding how the body works and what you need to do will lead to results.

3. **Execute:** Acting is more important than knowing. Once you have a clear vision and plan, it's time to achieve it.

HOW CAN YOU LIVE THIS OUT?

You've got this. It's not rocket science. Every chapter will share an idea to shape the way you think so you can make choices and take action. Each chapter then ends with three big ideas and three action steps. When you internalize a big idea or implement an action step, your life will get better. Don't look at this simply as losing weight. Rather, I am coaching you to a better life using fat loss as the tool. I am not a "weight-loss guy" but a life coach who went on a year-and-a-half journey to become a better me. I can help you do the same.

Yes, I want you to lose unwanted fat, but more importantly, I want you to have more energy to enjoy your life. Simply put, I want you to live better. Let's get after it!

24

DREAM AGAIN

The old man was dreaming about the lions.[1]

I felt stuck. I was tired. I lay in my bed with tear-filled eyes, full of pain and loss. This came out of nowhere, was unexpected and un-welcomed. I had finished reading The Old Man and the Sea, and the last line in the book struck me: "The old man was dreaming about the lions." This book captures the life story of a fisherman named Santiago, specifically his battle with a massive marlin. He miraculously catches the fish, but it's then devoured by sharks, ending in a total loss. Santiago lived a difficult life, but when things were hard, he dreamed about a time in his youth when he watched the lions of Africa playing by the ocean.

At first, I didn't understand why I was overcome by emotion. Then I realized, I teared up because I had lost the ability to dream. Life had worn me down, and I had accepted many life circumstances that now angered me. You would never know by looking from the outside that I was hurting on the inside. I was fighting the stresses and demands of life, dissatisfied that all my work didn't have a greater benefit and that many areas of life simply weren't going the way I wanted. This included unwanted weight gain and a sense of being out of control, often eating to manage stress. And the discontent was compounded by feelings of failure from a lack of self-discipline in working out.

CHOOSING TO DREAM AGAIN

In that moment on my bed, I chose to dream again. I chose to live differently and regain things I had lost. This decision changed the trajectory of my life. As I refocused, I realized one of the things holding me back was a lack of energy from progressive weight gain. It was clear that I needed to lose weight and increase my daily energy to truly enjoy life once again.

WHAT ABOUT YOU?

How would you feel with stronger muscles, less fat, and more energy? It's 100 percent possible to change your body. Ironically, the biggest battle is not physical but mental. If you can win in your mind, you will stay focused and motivated. The rest is simply practicing basic principles over time.

Our dream begins with a clear picture or vision in your mind. It will motivate your thoughts, words, actions, and behaviors to transform the way your body works and feels. Bottom line: your vision will bring focus and order to your life.

Imagine yourself thinner and with more energy. Picture watching your muscles grow, sensing more strength and confidence as your clothes become looser and others notice the change. Confidence grows as we look and feel better. People will sense positive growth as you regain control over what you eat and how you feel. Simple things anyone can do add up over time.

Take time to dream. Let current pain, lack of energy, and dissatisfaction drive you to seek something better. The more defined and vivid your dream, the stronger the motivation and clearer the path. Stop accepting things as life hands them to you. It's time to go on the offense and move forward. A clear vision and dream are starting points to a better reality. Paint a picture in your mind that will drive you to a better future.

BOTTOM LINE: YOU CAN DO THIS

Imagine how you would look and feel if you dropped that unwanted twenty, thirty, or more pounds. How much better would life be if you simply felt better and had more energy? How much more could you do? What would it be like to enjoy life again? I want to help get you there.

MY DREAM BROUGHT FOCUS

I spent years playing around with losing a few pounds here and there, but I didn't have a set destination, a clear picture in my head. Then it hit me. I wanted to weigh the same on my fiftieth birthday that I weighed at graduation. What graduation you ask? There were two. I graduated high school at 190 pounds, then gained to 226 in college to play football. I stopped playing college football after my second major knee surgery, focused more on fitness, and then weighed 190 pounds when I graduated with my master's degree at age twenty-five. At age forty-eight, I was back to weighing 226 pounds but with diminishing energy and increasing pains. It was then I dreamed of how life would change if I reached 190 pounds again.

I saw it: my goal was to weigh 190 pounds on my fiftieth birthday. Keep in mind, I didn't see this picture when I was feeling good and confident; it came into focus when I was fat and tired. Nobody was fat shaming me, but I felt bad about myself almost every day. Mentally, I was done. I didn't care about what anyone else thought. I needed to do it for me. I needed to feel better both in my body and my thoughts. I committed to my dream: weighing 190 on my fiftieth birthday.

VISION ORDERS YOUR ACTIONS

Once I had a vision of where I wanted to go, everything changed. Having some vague wishy-washy feeling of "wanting to be in shape" or "lose a couple of pounds" hadn't worked, but my clear vision and specific goal motivated me to get where I wanted to go. Honestly, just about everyone I know in their forties and fifties—and many other ages— want to "lose weight" or "feel better," but it rarely leads to real change. My transformation began with small, consistent changes and ended with an all-in effort for a couple of months. Every step was driven by a vivid picture, the dream I held in my mind.

CELEBRATE SMALL WINS

My new vision changed my actions, and I realized some wins physically and emotionally. Small changes repeated over time stopped the negative trend of gaining weight and losing energy and resulted in a gradual weight loss. I was finally trending in the right direction. Knowing I'd have to go harder at the end to ultimately reach my dream, I focused on building muscular strength and endurance as a strong foundation for future effort.

GETTING AFTER IT

Over time, action and vision feed each other. Vision informs how you order what you do. Doing the right things makes the vision clearer and more attainable over time. Setting a goal date forced me to move.

Before that, casual, slow progress was good but wasn't getting me to my goal fast enough. I increased effort, learned more about how my body works at fifty, and deciphered the changes in eating and exercise I wouldn't have had to make twenty—or even ten—years before.

SHIFT FROM "SHOULD DO" TO "MUST DO"

A clear goal shifted my thinking from something I "should do" to something I "must do." Everyone knows we should exercise and eat healthy but most of us simply don't do it. My dream caused a mental shift that made all the difference. My consistency and intensity increased exponentially. I made simple changes that I repeated over time. My "should go to the gym" become I "must go." "I shouldn't eat" that candy bar or drink that soda became "I won't."

When you allow your dream and vision to burn in your soul, many things others view as sacrifices become simple adjustments you feel proud to make as you chase your dream.

VISION OF A NEW LIFE

Let me be clear. My goal was not merely to lose a little weight. My dream was to live a different life: to drop forty pounds and keep it off; to live with more energy, passion, and fulfillment. My goal was not temporary deprivation but to live better for the next four to five decades. This mindset drove me forward.

CHOOSE TO WIN

Winning motivates me. I reached my goal because I turned my fitness and weight-loss process into a fight I resolved to win. Previously, I had been losing as I gained unwanted fat, lost daily energy, and watched my body deteriorate.

When I saw my declining energy and unwanted fat as "losing," it was game on. We are told to accept these realities as a normal part of aging, but I saw it as simply accepting defeat. I had to get it straight in my head first. Then I could make the daily decisions required to produce wins in my body.

IT STARTS AND FINISHES WITH YOUR DREAM

Nobody can dream for you. No one cares as much about how you feel and live as you do. Nobody has the ability to drive you to do or be something different. At the end of the day, you must motivate yourself to live better. You have to want it. Your dream is your goal, the finish line you are running toward. A new life chapter begins on the other side of that finish line, but you first have to run the race. When you have a clear picture in your mind, you are able to order your life to get there. Your dream functions like the destination in a GPS system, telling you what to do at every turn.

You can do it. After you have a clear picture of where you are going, the next step is to shift your mindset and stay focused on that dream.

BIG IDEAS

Learn to dream again.

Having a clear dream/vision changes everything.

Your vision determines your actions.

ACTION STEPS

Take the time to dream.

Celebrate small victories.

Let your dream motivate you to keep going.

SHIFT YOUR MINDSET

*Once your mindset changes, everything on the outside
will change along with it.* —STEVE MARABOLI [2]

I had the wrong mindset. Over time, I unintentionally adopted a losing mindset when it came to health and bodyweight. The saying goes, "If you fail to plan, you plan to fail." Essentially, for two decades or so, I had no plan to promote health. I went through life with my mind on autopilot regarding daily energy and bodyweight. Physically, I lived out losing strategies and behaviors. Before I could achieve my desired weight loss, I needed to shift my mindset.

Mindset: *an attitude, disposition, or mood; an intention or inclination* [3]

LET YOUR DREAM DRIVE YOUR MINDSET

My attitude, disposition, mood, and intention had been passive when it came to taking proper care of myself. Nobody intentionally gains unwanted weight or strives to have less energy, but if we are not purposely pursuing health and taking care of ourselves, it will happen.

With a clear dream and goal, I deliberately claimed a new mindset: a new attitude, disposition, intention, and inclination toward food, exercise, time management, and priorities. Life is a never-ending series of choices, and every choice results in a consequence, whether good or bad. When I chose to change my mindset, the consequence was a healthier life. If you want your life to go in a new direction, you must claim a new mindset.

WHERE DO I START WITH MY NEW MINDSET?

Get ready for some deep wisdom on how to start. Ready? Just start! Brilliant, right? Do something, do anything, but start. Own it. Take responsibility of every action and every bite of food—not in a weird way but in an intentional way. Walk up and down your stairs three times. Stand in front of the mirror and do twenty side bends; throw out the last three cookies and get angry at the cookies for making you fatter than you want to be. Feel something. Do something. Just start. Own it.

CLEAN AND CLEAR BEGINNING

One of the greatest determinants of reaching our goals is starting well. With your dream keeping you focused and your new mindset guiding you step-by-step, you are ready for a new start. If changed lifestyle is your goal, prepare mentally and physically. Reaching a goal requires a journey. A clear start and end goal are both extremely helpful and necessary. Our plan becomes our GPS. It knows the starting point and goal destination. It guides us there.

GET MENTALLY READY

Over the years, we've heard the phrase the "battlefield of the mind," meaning we win or lose challenges in our minds. Emotions and thoughts are incredibly powerful. They shape our actions. If our mindset is clear, we can win the outward battle. So, if our goal is to lose unwanted fat and feel better each and every day, we must first win the battle in our mind.

DAILY NEW BEGINNINGS

One way to stay focused is to look at each day as a new beginning and then resolve to "win" that day. If yesterday was good, awesome. Now win again today. If yesterday you slacked on exercising and made bad food choices, yesterday is gone. Focus on winning today. When we win each day, we build momentum and gain energy from our results and progress.

GET BACK ON THE WAGON

People are funny. If they mess up once in trying a new routine, they get frustrated, give up, and go back to the old destructive habit. But by looking at each day as a new beginning, you get a fresh start every twenty-four hours. If you have a bad day, just start again the next day. Your long-term results come from cumulative effects over time; results aren't dependent on one bad decision or day. It's like a batter who swung and missed; he needs to focus on the next pitch rather than dwelling on the strike. After you lose those unwanted pounds and have more energy, no one is going to know or care that you skipped a workout or ate a donut.

WINNING MINDSET FOCUSES ON WHAT MATTERS MOST

To change your life, you need to change your priorities. –Mark Twain[4]

One key to my success was a deliberate choice to enjoy life again. The weight-loss process allowed me, or possibly forced me, to refocus my entire life. One of the ways we keep our daily energy levels high is simply by enjoying life. The average person is too busy doing too many things to enjoy anything. Most of us are overbooked and undersatisfied. Essentially, we are not focused on the things that matter most. A focused life leads to greater fulfillment, more energy, and a better mindset.

BUILDING YOUR SOUL

Our soul is our mind, emotions, moods, and thought processes. It includes our intellect and mindset. It determines and holds all of who we are on the inside. Our entire mindset and quality of our lives flows out of our soul and spirit. If our soul is prospering, everything else will flow from that. If our soul is empty, depleted, or damaged, it will affect every aspect of our lives. Focusing time and energy on what matters most brings joy and allows us to do the most important things, which will bring the greatest results.

FEELING GOOD ABOUT WHAT YOU DO AFFECTS YOUR ENERGY AND BODYWEIGHT

If you are not focused on what matters most, you will eventually have less energy. This makes life and all you do more difficult. A cycle begins: low energy causes us to eat more (especially junk food for a "sugar rush"), which causes an insulin dump and stores fat, eventually returning us back to that low-energy level.

When we don't feel good, work becomes drudgery and even the things we love to do become a list of endless tasks. Losing weight became important to me because I didn't have the energy to enjoy my wife, children, friends, work, or even recreational fun. I became a working machine with no life. I had to stop making excuses, blaming people and life circumstances; instead, I made real, lasting changes—and that required a change in mindset.

DO EXERCISE OR ACTIVITY YOU LIKE

To maintain a continuous, active lifestyle and get to your desired fitness level, pick exercise and physical activities you enjoy. If you're someone who hates regimented exercise, focus on physical activities, such as walking your dog twice a day for half an hour, doing yard work, taking dance class, or pursuing other recreational hobbies. Some of these activities may not be as efficient as regimented exercise, but at the end of the day, movement is medicine; it all burns calories and builds muscle. Many roads can lead to transformation, so don't despair if you'll never be a gym rat.

SELF-DISCIPLINE MINDSET

Not a popular word these days, but self-discipline is one of your most powerful tools. Once you make the decision to be disciplined, it doesn't matter what you like or feel. You get after it. One of my greatest tools for losing forty pounds was old-fashioned self-discipline. For my final stretch, I committed to doing thirty minutes every day on the elliptical for the last fifty-one days of my weight loss. Game on. It didn't matter what I felt like or what I wanted to do instead. I was all in. This was the greatest factor to my success.

EAT HEALTHY FOODS YOU LIKE

Part of maintaining a positive mindset over time is enjoying the foods you eat. You will not stick to a diet of foods you don't like. Yes, you should cut out and minimize fried foods, junk food, and fast food, but you have to replace your old standbys with foods you like. One of the cool things about eating healthy is that your taste buds will become more sensitive. When you cut out fried, fatty, and sugary foods, you start to taste food more.

At the end of my weight loss, I hadn't drunk anything but water, black coffee, and fresh vegetable juice for about two months. One day, my eleven-year-old asked me if I wanted her to make tea for me, and I said yes. She makes a big deal out of it, so I couldn't say no.

She made chamomile tea and went through the whole process of heating the water in her little teapot, soaking the tea, adding blueberries, and then adding Splenda®. It seemed like the sweetest thing I had ever drunk. Also, fruit just became amazing because I had removed all sweets for two months. Part of maintaining a positive mindset over time is taking advantage of special moments like this.

Your mindset affects everything you do. Keeping your mindset focused and positive will keep progress moving forward. If you want to progress even faster, catch a little bit of attitude.

BIG IDEAS

Your mindset must be stronger than your obstacles.

Becoming fatigued is a process but so is gaining greater energy.

Regain control by planning your meals and exercise times.

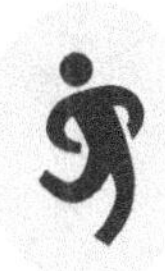

ACTION STEPS

Write or type out your goal weight and set a realistic date.

Purposely reject a constant state of fatigue as you
follow a plan to rejuvenate.

Purposely get motivated every day to make progress.
Every step brings you closer to your goal weight, increased energy,
and better overall health.

GET AN ATTITUDE

Winning isn't everything; it's the only thing. –Henry Sanders[5]

To reach my goal, I had to catch a nasty attitude—not toward people but toward the fat I wanted gone. I learned that the rate I lost fat was directly connected to my attitude. When I was focused on small changes and regular, steady workouts, I lost twenty-three pounds over about 14 months. I had a solid attitude while I steadily increased exercise and ate better. Along the way, when my attitude got lax, I gained a few pounds and had to get some attitude back. For the last seventeen pounds, I got aggressive toward exercise and food selection and timing. Bottom line was that weight loss was directly correlated to the aggressiveness of my attitude.

I NEEDED TO OVERCOME A LOUSY ATTITUDE

For years, I settled for less than my best. I neglected my body and ate wrong foods at wrong times. It added up. Denial or simply not caring ruled my attitude. But then frustration, regret, and even anger took hold as I realized my body was deteriorating. I needed significant and long-term change.

I was losing, and I knew it. Many times in life I beat others simply by working harder and having a better attitude. But here I was losing to myself. Year by year I slowly gained unwanted weight as my daily energy level decreased. When I focused for a short time, I lost a couple of pounds and increased my energy level, but life would happen, and the weight would return. Life kept getting a little bit harder year by year.

My feelings transitioned from a gnawing sense of possibility to full-blown ownership of the losing game I was playing. The choice stared me in the face like facing a kid who wanted to fight on the playground: would I fight or walk away? Walking away meant simply staying the course: make a few small changes, keep going to the gym two to three days a week, and tell myself I was okay. I could also compare myself to others who were in worse shape to convince myself I wasn't losing.

Fighting meant adjusting my attitude, changing my game plan, and making significant lifestyle changes. I knew that since it took about twenty years to get to this point, it would take time to get to where I wanted to be. But I took the challenge. I chose to win. I started with a nine-month game plan that ended up taking about sixteen months to complete. The first step was changing my attitude, which led to a solid decision to live differently. It took about nine to ten months for my body to get to a healthy place. Then it took two to three months of solid workouts and about three months of all-in, game-on lifestyle to truly change my life.

SLOW AND STEADY ATTITUDE

My original goal was to lose thirty-five pounds in thirty-five weeks, slow and steady at one pound per week. This attitude was good, especially as I transitioned from being out of shape to increased muscular strength and increased cardiovascular fitness. Adding fruits and vegetables while reducing junk food and fast food also helped the slow, steady loss. This built a strong foundation as I made more nourishing food choices in preparation to go harder to meet my goal.

INCREASINGLY AGGRESSIVE ATTITUDE

As my fitness increased through gaining strength and endurance, working out became a different activity. It went from feeling like work to being enjoyable and from drudgery to one of my favorite parts of the day. I went from loving junk food to scowling at cookies and ice cream. I went from feeling old to feeling like a brand-new person.

EXECUTE

I don't diet and exercise. I eat and train.[6]

Execution determines whether or not we will reach our goal. Executing is purposely following the details of our plan and making needed adjustments along the way. After creating the plan, working the plan is called *execution.*

Execute: to carry out; accomplish; to execute a plan or order[7]

Remember our three steps to reach a major life goal:
1. Dream
2. Plan
3. Execute

Dreaming occurs when we paint a picture in our mind of what we want to experience or live. This creates a clear vision of our goal. The next step is to *plan* the path we will take to move toward our dream/vision. To reach our destination, the final step is to *execute* our plan.

Execution occurs when we put in the work. We can talk all day about how we need to build muscle, burn fat, and eat right, but the work must be executed according to the plan if we want results. The more powerful the vision, the better the plan. Proper execution of the plan will help us reach our goal. We must decide how and when we will work out and what and when we will eat. Then we must stick to the plan and make needed adjustments to reach our goals.

YOU ARE IN CONTROL

Attitude determines everything. Every day, you choose what you eat and how much you exercise. You are in control. Life may be tough; you may have limited resources and time. Welcome to reality. Even so, you still call the shots for your body. No one is force-feeding you cookies and potato chips or forbidding you to exercise.

EATING HUMBLE PIE

The process humbled me. It was hard to have an aggressive attitude and be humble at the same time, but learning this balance taught me so much about myself and life. I needed to put down my pride, my knowledge, and my ego. I had to ask questions and take painful criticism, but through it all, I grew.

For the last eight weeks of my journey, I shaved my head and my beard. I put myself in boot camp. I didn't like it; my wife and kids didn't like it either, but I was going somewhere. My beard had been hiding my double chin. My hair was short but now bald—and bald was never my goal. It felt naked and vulnerable, but it was a statement to the world that my life was shifting. My attitude said *all in*.

Part of this was also timing. I was turning fifty. And it was the be-ginning of a new decade: 2020. I was coming out of the hardest decade of my life. It was the perfect storm, and I took the fight and won with a winning game plan and discipline. Honestly, it was more fun than pain-ful and turned into a life-changing experience.

SIMPLE

At the end of the day, my process was simple. It was easy to under-stand and follow, and my goal is to share it with others. Yesterday is gone, and you can't get it back. You only have today. If you take care of today, tomorrow will take care of itself. Right now, you're on the play-ground, and the bully is staring you down. You have a choice: will you walk away, or will you fight? It's that simple.

To reach my goal, I needed to change my attitude. I needed to ex-amine the direction of my life and consider the outcome if I continued on the current path. I saw the unwanted fat as an unwanted guest and enemy of my best life. When I developed a negative attitude toward fat, my life momentum shifted to a different direction.

Weight loss doesn't begin in the gym with a dumb bell; it starts in your head with a decision. –Toni Sorenson[8]

At my core, I am a passionate and even aggressive guy. This trait has been evident many times in my life: in sports, in education and career goals, and in pursuit of my interests. Passionate is who I am at my core, but I had lost my edge. This realization has helped me not judge oth-ers. If I can lose my edge, anyone can. The opposite is also true. If I can regain my edge from my lowest point, then so can you.

EYE OF THE TIGER

The series of *Rocky* movies shaped my mindset as a youth. *Rocky* tells the story of a young boxer in Philadelphia whose future doesn't look promising. He is an average club fighter trying to survive. But then he gets a chance to fight Apollo Creed, the world champ, because Apollo needs an opponent at the last minute. The story is in the tradition of David and Goliath. Rocky loses their first fight by decision, but it is a huge victory because he didn't get knocked out, and he also badly hurt the champ at the end. He came back in *Rocky II* to beat Apollo Creed for the title.

Rocky III begins a few years later in Rocky's life. This previously poor, low-class, and uneducated but hungry street guy is now living in a mansion after winning a bunch of fights. Success, comfort, and excessive confidence have replaced passion. Then along comes a young, hungry guy named Clubber Lang, played by Mr. T. He totally destroys Rocky and knocks him out. The plot thickens as Apollo Creed, Rocky's old nemesis, comes to train him. Apollo begins by bringing Rocky to the local gym where he grew up. When they get there, they take a look at all the young fighters who have a glint in their eye. Apollo says, "Do you see it?" Rocky asks, "See what?" Apollo replies, "The eye of the tiger." Apollo means they all have the look of a hungry tiger about to go in for the kill.

Apollo then humbly admits that the reason Rocky beat him was that he himself lost the eye of the tiger. Apollo Creed was always a much better boxer but Rocky was simply hungrier when they met in the ring. Apollo told Rocky that the reason he had lost to Clubber Lang was because, over time, he too had lost the eye of the tiger. I was losing my weight battle because I lost my hunger to be in shape and to be my best.

I LOST IT ALL

I lost the eye of the tiger. I lost my swag. Real talk is that I spent the last fifteen years getting my butt kicked. I was working eighty to one hundred hours a week and trying to raise four kids. It seemed as if everything and the kitchen sink was thrown at me. I faced every emotion imaginable over the years: exhaustion, anger, sadness, hopelessness, and being overwhelmed. I made it through so much but somehow lost my hunger and got sloppy. I no longer had the eye of the tiger—more like eye of the crybaby.

I HAD TO TURN THINGS AROUND

I needed to get in the right mental space to succeed. Weight gain and weight loss is more than eating right and exercising. Everyone knows that if they exercise more and eat better, they will lose weight. But a certain attitude is required to see it through.

In the movie, Rocky went back with Apollo to South Central, Los Angeles, to train in a no-frills gym with no-frills guys because he had to regain the eye of the tiger. Before I started the weight-loss program, I determined to get control of and strengthen some other key parts of my life, like my relationship with my wife, kids, and friends, my career, and our finances. When those areas no longer felt out of control, I could direct my focus solely on getting strong and healthy and regaining the eye of the tiger.

THE RIGHT ATTITUDE GETS RESULTS

If you can get your attitude right, everything else becomes easier. My success came when my mind was right, and my passion came from within. In the world of motivation, two main forces motivate us: extrinsic and intrinsic motivation.

EXTRINSIC VS. INTRINSIC MOTIVATION

Extrinsic motivation comes from the outside. For example, when you were doing something wrong as a kid and your parent walked in the room and you stopped, that was extrinsic motivation at work. The desire to stop wasn't from within yourself. In fact, you were choosing to do the wrong thing. But when the fear of punishment came in the room, you changed your behavior. How many times do children return to the same wrong activity once the parent leaves?

In terms of weight loss, friends or society remarking on your extra weight will motivate you for a little while, but once that negative pressure isn't there, you will probably go back to bad or lazy habits. On the job, you have probably worked with that guy who cuts every corner until the boss is present, when he then switches to working hard and kissing up—until the boss leaves.

Intrinsic motivation, in contrast, comes from within and is not dependent on who is watching. The guy at work who shows up early and is geeked out to work hard every day is intrinsically motivated. The slacker is motivated extrinsically by the boss's presence, but the go-getter is motivated from within. As a business owner, I am always looking for people who are intrinsically motivated because they are driven from within to get things done. They have the eye of the tiger. It doesn't matter what's thrown at them, they are ready to tackle it.

YOU HAVE TO WANT IT

This is not easy. You have to want to lose weight and keep it off. Once I got that eye of the tiger back, I wasn't stressed out about food choice or taking time to go to the gym. I went from dreading the elliptical for twenty minutes to feeling like something was missing if I didn't do it for an hour. When my attitude changed, a hunger within me gave me control over my thoughts and actions.

I HAD TO DO IT FOR MYSELF

Let me be honest. I realized that whether or not my wife was attracted to me or what others thought about my weight was not sufficient motivation. Once I got to a point where I didn't focus on what my friends, coworkers, wife, kids, or anyone else thought, my attitude shifted. I regained intrinsic motivation, which resulted in a sense of freedom and empowerment.

I started going through life like a hot knife through soft butter. I easily trampled everything that once seemed tedious and draining. Things that stressed me out were now child's play. It wasn't the weight loss that changed my attitude; it was my attitude change that drove the weight loss.

SHUT OUT THE NOISE

My last bit of advice on staying motivated is to shut out the noise and negative comments of others. When I told people I was going to lose thirty-five pounds, many told me I didn't need to lose that much; they warned me "not to get too skinny" and discouraged me from going to the gym so frequently. I ended up losing forty pounds, and it was amazing how almost everyone shut up when I posted my fifty-year-old flex on Facebook. Of course, some people criticized that too, saying I was arrogant and showing off. I smiled because I posted it for me because I felt good about it. It wasn't for them.

ATTITUDE AND OUR THREE MAIN GOALS

Remember our three main goals to drop unhealthy and unwanted fat:

1. Build muscle
2. Burn fat
3. Eat right

Did you know you can catch an attitude to build muscle, burn fat, and eat right? When my attitude changed and got more aggressive, things just got easier. I went from thinking, *I have to go to the gym* (hear the whining) to, *"Man, I wish I had more time at the gym!"* I got excited about doing more reps on a machine to build muscle or increase my time on the elliptical or take an extra walk to burn more fat. I felt progress with every good food choice. My attitude shift changed my actions from drudgery and deprivation to passionate progress. Simply put, my winning attitude caused me to win.

BIG IDEAS

You must develop a winning attitude ("the eye of the tiger") to make powerful progress.

Sustainable motivation must come from within (intrinsic motivation).

Be a humble student. Keep going and keep learning.

ACTION STEPS

Check your attitude and make needed changes.

Purposely learn and study how the body works.

Train your mind to purposely choose healthy foods
and increase daily activity.

JUST GET STARTED

One of our biggest problems is not that we don't know what to do but that we don't do it. –Jack Redmond

To lose weight, all I needed to do was what I already knew I was supposed to. I knew this stuff. I spent my teen years reading every magazine and book on weightlifting I could get my hands on. I went to the gym six days a week for years and then spent many more years going at least three to five days per week. I have had classes on physiology, kinesiology, nutrition, and fitness on undergraduate and graduate levels, including the number one-rated graduate school in the nation, Teacher's College at Columbia University. Even if I don't "know it all," I probably come pretty close on understanding the basics of fat loss. But to lose weight, I had to do what I already knew. I had to stop making excuses and just get started.

MAKE A DECISION AND GO

When's the best time to start? Today! Just about everyone on planet earth knows that if they eat less and exercise more, they will lose weight. No PhD required for that knowledge. Yes, I know fitness is more complicated than that, but to get started, you only need the basics: eat better, move more. Said differently, go for a walk and trade that Twinkie for a carrot. You get it.

NO ONE IS FAT IN AMERICA BECAUSE OF
LACK OF INFORMATION

You can literally go online and learn how to lose weight. As long as you choose reputable sources, you can get free workouts, eating plans, and wellness information. We have more knowledge available than any other time in history. So why are more people obese and overweight than ever? Remember, what we do impacts us more than the flood of knowledge and information available to us. Yes, we want to obtain the best knowledge and techniques, but the person who can grasp the basics and do them will succeed.

In fact, if you don't want to read the rest of this book, I can help you in one sentence. Ready? Every day, walk three miles, do one set of push-ups until you fatigue, eat three healthy meals, and substitute water, fruit, and vegetables for soda, juices, and junk food. There you go. This one sentence will change your life. But you probably already knew all that. This is about behavior, people.

MY BEHAVIOR GOT ME FAT

I played sports and worked out my whole life. I have an undergraduate degree in health and physical education with a specialization in athletic training. I did my graduate work in applied physiology and nutrition at Columbia University and did an internship with the Kansas City Chiefs in the NFL. All this said, my knowledge didn't keep me from getting fat.

I ignored what I knew and neglected my health. I made excuses and relied on my past physical shape and accomplishments. I knew my lack of exercise and my food choices were not the best, but I ignored the facts. But 190 became 200, then 205, then 215. I bounced back and forth half-heartedly. It wasn't until I hit 225 and eventually 228 that I determined to change my behaviors.

I WAS GETTING BETTER AT GETTING FATTER

Don't laugh, but the first thing that happened when I committed to losing thirty-five pounds was that I gained three pounds. You may be chuckling because that's funny, or you may be chuckling because you have shared my experience. As we age, our body changes, and if we just keep eating the same way and don't exercise enough, the weight seems to show up. It becomes easier to gain weight as our metabolism slows down. *Metabolism* is how fast your body burns calories. When I was younger, I could literally eat anything at any time of day without gaining weight. Let's just say this is no longer the case.

Growing up, I was on the short and skinny side—not a problem except that I wanted to be a football player. So, from the age of fourteen to twenty-two, I force-fed myself and lifted weights. So, after about ten years of eating six or more times a day and lifting weights anywhere from three to six days a week, I tipped the scales at 226 pounds. This was great for a college middle linebacker because most of it was muscle. When I was done playing football, I stopped lifting weights so much and got a mountain bike. Riding twenty to thirty miles a day, I got down to 190 pounds. Then over the last twenty years the weight crept up until I hit 226 again.

THE CURRENT 226 WAS NOT THE GOOD 226

It might have been the same weight, but I had a totally different body composition. Though I can't cite a body composition test, I suspect I had thirty pounds less muscle and thirty pounds more fat. When I took my shirt off at my weightlifting 226, the college girls said, "Ooh." If I took my shirt off at middle-age 226, college girls would have probably said, "Ewww." Same weight, different body composition.

When we look at health, weight is not the only factor. One of the key things we want to do is increase our muscle mass and decrease our body fat percentage. It's simple: the more muscle we have and the less body fat, the healthier we are. Muscle is active tissue that burns calories, supports our bones and joints, and helps us feel stronger and more confident. Fat is inactive tissue that stresses our body, including our heart, lungs, and joints. So, my extra weight was like carrying around a thirty-five-pound backpack all day. No wonder I felt tired.

SMALL BEHAVIORS ADD UP

Many of us don't get on the right path because we think we need to be on an extreme path to lose weight. My first goal is to help you see that losing weight can be simple. Small changes add up over time. I didn't gain my extra thirty-five pounds by doing anything extreme. One pound of fat is thirty-five hundred calories. If, over the course of one month, I ate an extra five hundred calories on seven out of thirty days, I would have gained one pound in that month. Do that for twelve months and you just gained twelve pounds of fat. Little changes add up over time. Imagine you overate five hundred calories on only seven different days over the course of four months. That would add up to three pounds in a year. That would be thirty-six pounds from age thirty-six to forty-eight You can see how easy it is to add twenty or thirty pounds over the course of a couple of decades.

DEFINING AND USING CERTAIN TERMS

Throughout the book, I will use certain terms, definitions, and standards to make points and share broad principles that anyone can put into practice. The topics of exercise and nutrition consistently bring up debate, anecdotal stories, and personal preferences. There are many approaches and schools of thought. But I wrote this book to help the average person implement solid physiological and nutritional principles to lose fat and increase energy. So, let's start with the basics.

Calorie: a unit of energy or heat variously defined. The calorie was originally defined as the amount of heat required at a pressure of one standard atmosphere to raise the temperature of one gram of water 1° Celsius.[9]

one pound of fat = approximately thirty-five hundred extra calories of stored as fat

Because thirty-five hundred calories equals about one pound (0.45 kilogram) of fat, it's estimated that you need to burn about thirty-five hundred calories to lose one pound.[10]

SHOULD I COUNT CALORIES?

If counting helps you, then, yes, count your calories. But I don't believe you have to. I use numbers to illustrate behavioral changes and often say, "It's math," because over time, if you burn more calories than you eat, you will lose weight. I personally have never counted calories, but if that helps you stay focused, then do it. I think in broader terms and promote better food choices to eliminate empty calories. For in-stance, if I eat that candy bar, I will have to run three miles to burn it off, so I opt for an apple and glass of water.

Some people get all geeked out with numbers and feeling diligent motivates them, but simple is best for me. It's your race to run and win, so use these principles but make them work in your life.

BEHAVIOR AND OUR THREE MAIN GOALS

We will get into details as we progress, but I know many people are action oriented and want to do something. Below are behavioral recommendations to get you started with our basic three goals:

1. **Build muscle:** Do resistance training at least two to three days a week (lift weights, calisthenics, machines, etc.). Start slow and build up over time.

2. **Burn fat:** Add cardiovascular exercise, such as walking, jogging, cycling, swimming, etc., for at least twenty minutes three to six days a week. If you are in good shape, you can do high intensity interval training (HIIT) workouts.

3. **Eat right:** Make healthy food choices and eat three meals a day (unless purposely fasting). Snack on and increase fruits and vegetables.

BEHAVIOR DRIVES PROGRESS

It's behavior that makes the difference. The guy with the third-grade education who goes to the gym every day is going to do better than the guy with a PhD in physiology or kinesiology who sits on his couch and eats donuts.

The more you learn and apply, the better. If you need more information before starting, that's fine. Keep reading. But no matter where you are, start. If nothing else, you can start a purposeful walking program.

LET'S WALK

Walking is the best medicine. —HIPPOCRATES[11]

Walking is simple. Anyone can do it, and walking will help you lose weight. No matter the methods of exercise you use, walking should be part of the program. Over time, we have gone from walking everywhere to riding buses, driving cars, and taking elevators and escalators instead of stairs. With each technological advancement, we have unconsciously cut out much of the activity that used to happen naturally. Remember that losing weight is simple math. If we eat the same number of calories but increase activity, such as walking, those burned calories will add up, and we will eventually lose unwanted fat.

WALKING IS SIMPLE

Unless injured or suffering a medical condition that prohibits it, anyone can walk. You have no excuses. Increasing the distance you walk increases the calories you burn. You don't have to learn anything new or practice a technique or skill. You simply have to walk more. By increasing distance and pace, you can also increase fat burning.

WALKING AS A WORKOUT

Walking is cardiovascular exercise, and fat is burned most efficiently through cardiovascular exercise. Fat breakdown is a chemical process in which fat is broken down through combining with oxygen in the midst of the energy demand of exercise:

$$O_2 + C_{58}H_{12}O_6 \rightarrow CO_2 + H_2O + energy[12]$$

Oxygen combined with a fat molecule during exercise causes fat to be broken down into carbon dioxide and water while simultaneously releasing energy to meet the body's need for fuel to perform the exercise. Breathing is increased. The inhale supplies the body with needed oxygen for this chemical reaction to take place, and the exhale rids the body of carbon dioxide. Water produced in this process is utilized within the body for different functions. Basically, the longer you exercise, the greater the demand for energy and ongoing oxygen supply, which leads to more fat breakdown.

Knowing this equation motivated me to go longer every time I stepped on the elliptical. I understood that the longer I went and the more energy I put out, both oxygen intake and energy usage would increase, resulting in more fat burned.

WALKING CAN BE MAINTAINED FOR EXTENDED PERIODS

Walking can get us into fat-burning range while allowing us to maintain the activity for longer periods. It's simple: increased time in fat-burning range means an increased amount of fat burned. Walking is also low impact, meaning it can be maintained without causing injury, so it's a great option if a person has an injury that keeps them from doing higher-impact, more rigorous forms of exercise.

WHAT IF WALKING IS DIFFICULT?

Some people have difficulty walking even short distances due to injury, illness, or carrying too much weight. With all exercise, please follow your doctor's guidelines and don't do anything to further injure yourself or cause illness to flare. But the vast majority of people can walk without increasing injury. The longer and farther you go, the greater the benefit. So, start today.

DIFFERENT WAYS TO WALK OFF WEIGHT

1. Set a time each day for a twenty-minute (or more) walk. Make it your routine.

2. Deliberately park your car farther than normal and use stairs instead of elevators.

3. Take a walk break at work.

4. Turn your walks into workouts. By increasing your pace, walking up hills, or hiking, you can add distance and intensity.

WHY I HIKE

I hate running. I don't like it and probably never will, but I love to hike. My favorite hike is a little over three miles, and I would hit this trail every day if I had the time. But you probably couldn't pay me to walk or run three miles every day. Do what you love, and you'll do it more often.

Being outside also has health benefits. Sunshine increases vitamin D production. The fresh air, change of scenery, and quiet solitude all add up to a physically, emotionally, and spiritually beneficial experience. Hiking is basically walking but in a beautiful outdoor setting—and that makes a difference to me. Stress reduction is an added benefit for many.

Hiking also seems easier on my joints. Walking or jogging on the concrete increases impact, and the repetitive motion can aggravate or cause injury. With hiking, each step is different, so the body has to adjust. This brings more muscles into activation and more evenly applies the impact and stress to different parts of your body to reduce overuse injuries.

I deliberately clean out my body when I hike or exercise by drinking a lot of water. I look at it this way: the more I sweat and take in water, the more I am flushing out my body. Drinking water, sweating, and urinating cleanse your body and make it healthier. Purposeful behaviors add up over time.

TAKE CONTROL

You have control and can decide to build muscle, burn fat, and eat right each and every day. Every healthy choice benefits you, so the more healthy choices and actions you take, the greater the benefit. Even if you are still learning, you know enough by now to make progress that adds up over time. Feel hopeful about every healthy food choice and every workout, knowing that when you keep the progress going over time, the benefits will add up. The benefits start as soon as you begin. Don't overcomplicate it; just get started.

BIG IDEAS

Behavior is more important than knowledge.

Simple changes add up over time.

Everyone can walk (unless they have a physical limitation), so walk—the more, the better.

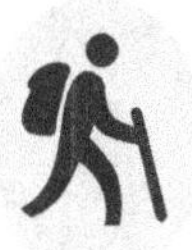

ACTION STEPS

Build the habit of writing down your behavioral goals
(i.e., lose five pounds this month, go to the gym Monday/Wednesday/
Saturday, drink sixty-four ounces of water daily).

Write grocery lists that include fruits, vegetables, and lean meats.
Exclude junk food and stick to your list at the store.

Purposely take steps: park farther away than necessary, use the stairs
instead of the elevator, and plan daily walks.

64

EMBRACE THE GRIND

*My confidence comes from knowing I do the right things in my life.
I do the right things in the gym. I do the right things all together.*[13]
—*"The King of the Grind," Daniel Cormier*
former Light Heavyweight and
Heavyweight World UFC Champion

To reach my weight loss goal, I needed to gradually build my exercise consistency and intensity over time while diligently making solid food choices. I had to "undo" unwanted weight gain that resulted from consistently making unwise food choices and not exercising. While you may think no one "diligently" makes bad food choices or "purposely" doesn't work out, I define my past behaviors that way. To achieve and maintain my goals, I needed to be consistent in both eating right and exercising.

It's not a quick fix. You must grind. *Grind* means you work hard each and every day until you get things done. It means being willing to work your butt off in ways most others won't to achieve things others never will. It's not complicated and doesn't require special talent. "To grind" simply requires consistent, purposeful, and aggressive effort. Anyone can wake up and grind.

I remember an overweight man who walked by my office window with his golden retriever every day. Over the course of months, he went from a guy wearing baggy clothes and hiding his body to walking without a shirt. After more time, you could see his abdominal muscles. I don't know anything else about this man, but I watched his transformation in real time. I can't speak to what he ate or what else he did, but the one thing I know is that he walked—a lot. He grinded, and I saw his body transform. No special talent was needed. He just went out every day and got it done.

If you will walk, jog, or go to the gym regularly, you will see positive results. Physiology works according to predictable principles. If you are willing to work hard to burn extra calories (grind), you will achieve results.

DANIEL CORMIER

Daniel Cormier was an Olympic wrestler and a two-weight UFC MMA World Champion at 205 pounds and heavyweight. Compared to many opponents, he is shorter and not as muscular, yet he was undefeated as a heavyweight for years but chose to cut forty pounds to compete at 205 pounds.

At forty pounds lighter, he won the light heavyweight title. Later, he moved back up to win the heavyweight title and simultaneously held both championships. This had never been done before or after.

Mixed martial arts (MMA) combines boxing, wrestling, karate, judo, and jiu-jitsu all at the same time. You can punch, kick, knee, flip, wrestle, twist arms or legs, and even use different chokeholds on your opponent. You win either by points for successful technique, by knocking people out, or by causing them to tap out due to pain or a chokehold. It is an incredibly challenging sport, and Cormier has had incredible success.

Cormier became one of the best fighters in the history of MMA. What is his secret? He is the "king of the grind." He simply out works, out trains, and out prepares others. If he can grind his way to be the captain of the United States Olympic wrestling team and a simultaneous two-division UFC champion, I knew I could grind away thirty-five pounds of cheeseburgers and bowls of late-night ice cream.

CLEAR CHOICE: MUST DO

One of my key motivators was a YouTube clip explaining the difference between "should do" and "must do." Its message is that when we label things as "should do," we leave room for another priority to bump it out of our focus and schedule. If we label it a "must do" with conviction, it will get the attention it needs to get done. Once you are locked in on a "must do," it will get done, and you'll reach more goals.

PEACE OF MIND

Once clearly defined, must dos bring peace. When I understand what I *must* do, I don't have to worry or stress. I only need to execute the plan. I already have it figured out, so I know the steps to walk it out. You get rid of all of the "ifs" and "maybes." The it-would-be-nice type of thinking is gone. You have your must do. So, grind.

GRIND = PROGRESS

The grind gives you progress, and progress is motivating, encouraging you to grind one more day, then one more week. The grind and progress feed each other and propel you toward your goals. Everything shifts when you embrace the grind; your goal becomes a mission.

In my weight-loss efforts, I slowly lost twenty-three pounds in a little over a year, but when I put myself in a two-month boot camp, I was all in. The last seventeen pounds flew off. I made the choice to do the elliptical every day from January 1 to February 20 for at least thirty minutes. During this fifty-one-day period, thirty minutes became thirty-five, then forty, and then a full-out sixty minutes at a time. As I embraced the grind, I saw more progress. As I saw progress, I pushed even harder. Everything changed.

I DIDN'T GIVE MY BODY A CHOICE

I knew what I was doing. I gave my body no choice but to burn fat. By building muscle, burning fat, and eating right, my body had no choice. Remember, physiology operates according to predictable principles. I ate well enough to get the needed nutrition and then went after it to burn the fat. Commitment to the grind also heightens focus in other areas.

THE RIPPLE EFFECT

After spending thirty to sixty minutes on the elliptical, I wasn't willing to sabotage that work with bad food choices. Choosing the grind with my workout disciplined my food choices. Other benefits included increased energy and visible physical change. After three weeks of my boot camp, and for the following month, everywhere I went, people commented on my weight loss. Such encouragement was highly motivational.

YOU CAN DO THIS

Remember, it's math. I knew that if I got on the elliptical every day,

I would make progress. If you eat the same exact food but do more cardio, you will burn fat. If you combine better food choices with careful timing of meals, you will lose even more. My favorite thing about this is that anyone can do it. It's a simple choice repeated. With each repetition of going to the gym and eating right, the results accumulate. Calories burned will add up and deplete your fat storage. Every time we build muscle, burn fat, and eat right, we move forward to our goals of having less fat and more energy.

MINDSET OF GRIND AND PERSEVERANCE

Perseverance: *Steady persistence in a course of action, a purpose, a state, etc., especially in spite of difficulties, obstacles, or discouragement.*[14]

Perseverance may be the most important trait a person needs to lose weight. If the grind is commitment to ongoing daily intensity, then perseverance is commitment to the long-term maintenance of the grind.

Losing weight is a marathon, not a sprint. A sprinter runs a short distance as fast as they can. Sprinters are impressive to watch, but even the best sprinters in the world will max out around four hundred meters as the body fatigues. This is generally considered the maximum distance a person can sprint.

The opposite of a sprint is a marathon, a 26.2-mile race that takes hours to complete and must be run at a much slower pace than a sprint. Due to the distance and the time, a marathon runner must master perseverance.

PERSEVERANCE REQUIRES ONGOING EFFORT

My goal of losing thirty-five pounds meant burning 122,500 calories more than I ate. I ended up losing forty pounds: 140,000 calories of fat. This required ongoing effort over time (aka perseverance). Perseverance can be applied to exercise and eating patterns. It can keep you moving forward when injured. The effort and energy must continue week after week and month after month.

PERSEVERANCE PUSHES THROUGH PAIN AND FRUSTRATION

When I signed up to lose thirty-five pounds, I didn't sign up for injuries. But in the process, I hurt my back twice, sprained muscles in both my big toes, had knee pain, hip pain, and pinched nerves in my neck several times. But I pushed through the pain both physically and mentally to stay focused on the end goal.

For me, frustration is painful. While losing this weight, I often had to work many long and late hours, which means I sometimes had to drink coffee or eat more food to keep going. My joke, which is not a joke, is that I have one wife, four kids, and three jobs. My landlord, boss, and people paying me to complete book projects and speak at their events didn't care that was trying to lose weight.

Life periodically intervened as I sought to lose the weight. I had to be realistic about my situation and keep the big picture in mind. I wanted to be the boss and bang it out to impress the world, but at times, I was less impressive than I would have liked. But even with setbacks, I kept going. Perseverance pushes through frustration.

PERSEVERANCE IN TIMES OF LOW CONFIDENCE

Here's a fun one. We must keep grinding when we have low confidence, when we feel like we can't, or when we fear it's more likely we will fail than succeed. When we feel like a failure or, even worse, when are truly failing in our efforts, we must continue to persevere. I went on a mission trip to Nicaragua, and they fed us well. One of the younger guys sent the team a message that he lost twelve pounds on the trip. I texted back that I found six to seven pounds of it. How do you gain weight on a mission trip? Somehow, I managed.

My goal of maintaining or losing weight on this trip was a failure. I could have given up or wallowed in my lapse. Instead, I persevered. We must keep going in spite of our emotions or even our reality. The only way to fail is to quit trying. We must persevere. We do that by waking up every day and grind.

BIG IDEAS

For faster and lasting progress, embrace the grind.

A mental shift takes place when you are all in.
Exercise and proper eating become lifestyle norms.

Anyone can do this, so make the decision to move forward.
Don't look back, even when you face stress or injury.

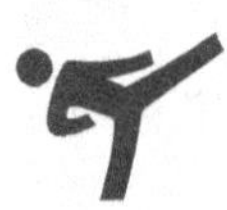

ACTION STEPS

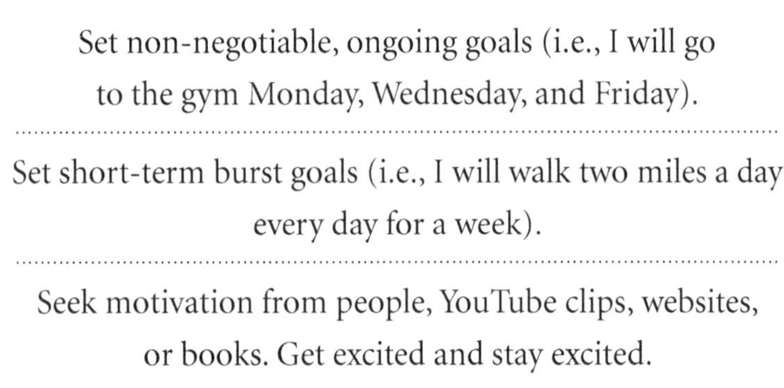

Set non-negotiable, ongoing goals (i.e., I will go
to the gym Monday, Wednesday, and Friday).

Set short-term burst goals (i.e., I will walk two miles a day
every day for a week).

Seek motivation from people, YouTube clips, websites,
or books. Get excited and stay excited.

REJECT NORMAL

If you are always trying to be normal,
you will never know how amazing you can be.
—MAYA ANGELOU [15]

To be healthy, to be my best, I had to reject "normal." Getting fat, having the dad bod, and maturing (aka getting a belly) are all considered normal. Even though I was overweight by all medical charts, many still came to me to learn how they could get fit—"like me." If feeling tired and out of shape is considered normal, I don't want to be normal. Instead, I want to help people who are overweight feel better and have more energy.

Every five years or so, I have experienced noticeable physical changes, along with the weight gain. As you get older, the changes may be more profound. I knew I couldn't totally stop the effects of aging, but I wanted to fight the energy decline and weight gain that was gaining momentum. I refused to hide behind the excuse that these things are normal and have to be accepted. As the weight came off, my daily energy level greatly increased. I learned that rejecting normal released power.

THE DOWNSIDE OF MODERN LIVING

Modern life has many benefits. For most of human history, simple survival was a struggle. Finding, growing, or killing food took great effort and was not always successful. In fact, historically, the only over-weight people were the rich as they had means to buy excessive food. In America today, many poor people are overweight; this is a new phenomenon. I recently saw a Facebook meme comparing poor starving people in Africa with poor overweight Americans. The meme said, "How can you be so poor and so fat at the same time?" Poor people are often overweight because unhealthy foods are cheaper. Many also lack sufficient exercise.

Modern farming and food distribution supply more to eat. We also have medicine to help us when we make ourselves sick from unhealthy, excessive food consumption. Cholesterol medicine and heart procedures (like stints and bypasses) greatly extend life. These advancements are blessings but don't fully address the decline in energy, excessive fat storage, and myriad physical problems caused by overeating.

On November 19, 2018, I stepped on the scale and weighed 225 pounds. Overall, I was healthy and in better shape than many of my peers, but honestly, I was overweight and on a slippery slope. At my last doctor's visit, my heart rate was in the sixties and my blood pressure was 110/70 or so. If I put on the right clothes, people told me I was fit. The reality is that, overall, our society is overweight, so perhaps I did appear to be an acceptable weight by comparison.

When I did a little research, I found that as a six-foot man, my ideal weight is about 180 pounds. I was forty-five pounds overweight but probably still more fit than about 90 percent of my modern-day peers. I'm not trying to judge, but our society as a whole is not as healthy as it could be. It might be normal, but how can carrying around forty-five pounds of extra fat be good for you?

DO I HAVE TO ACCEPT THIS?

No, we don't have to accept unwanted weight gain and low energy as normal. Over the previous years, when I spoke about my need to lose weight, many told me I didn't. But I knew my body and felt the increased weight and decreased energy. I wanted to be strong and vibrant for myself and my family. I wanted to live out my life with purpose.

I travel annually to Nicaragua and India to help the poorest of the poor and do leadership trainings with those who serve them in their communities. I want to be doing this when I am eighty and ninety years old, but that won't happen if I don't have the health and energy to do it.

FIFTY POUNDS OF FAT REVELATION

One day, when I weighed around 226 or 228 pounds, I was at the gym. I had been lifting pretty steadily, but honestly, I was nowhere near as strong as I once was. I began lifting weights in junior high school at my house, and in friends' garages. Then, in my freshman year in high school, I discovered the weight room, which became my second home for the next four years.

As I thought about cutting down to 190, one of my rationales was that I was stronger at 190 than at 225. While in the gym, I thought about how muscle is what makes you strong; fat is just there. So, if I was stronger at 190 than at 225, I probably had more muscle at 190. Then I thought about the details of lifting weights and remembered that when I was a 175-pound junior in high school, I was benching 250 pounds and squatting around 350 and deadlifting over 300 pounds.

I realized I was stronger at 175 than 225, which basically means I had more muscle at 175 than at 225, so I was walking around with fifty pounds of unnecessary fat. This was troublesome. I thought about it, and my mind raced. I kept saying, "I have fifty pounds of fat." Wow. This was an unwanted and painful revelation. I knew I needed to take this seriously, especially because it was only getting worse. But don't forget, I was well within what society was telling me was normal. Simply put, we must reject normal.

WE DON'T HAVE TO ACCEPT NORMAL

My goal is to help you live better. Too many people have low energy and lack zeal for life, or they are simply tired all the time. If the average guy is walking around with thirty to fifty extra pounds, is it any wonder he feels tired? The extra weight also stresses the heart and joints. I had pain in some of my joints when I was heavier and not working out. Why should we walk around tired and in pain when we don't have to?

We live in a society where we can easily gain the knowledge of weight loss or sign up for a local gym that has all the equipment we need for as little as ten dollars a month. We also have plentiful sources of healthy food. Simply put, we have everything we need, but we must take advantage of what is available.

NOT ABOUT PERFECTION

I will never have the body I had twenty years ago or wow anyone with my chiseled physique. I'm not twenty. But this is about being better, not perfect. I am not trying to impress anybody. Rather, I want to be healthy and the best me.

NOT ABOUT BEING ON ALL KINDS OF MEDICINE

I am not against medicine. In fact, I am grateful for the United States' medical system. But I don't want to be on medicines unnecessarily. My doctor had been suggesting cholesterol-lowering medicine for a couple of years. I said no because I don't have high cholesterol due to a medical condition. My cholesterol is too high because I have been undisciplined in how I eat. In fact, when I started taking fish oils, ate oatmeal for breakfast daily, and juiced vegetables and fruits, my cholesterol dropped by sixty points.

Normal would say take the medicine and keep eating whatever you want. In fact, that's what the doctor told me I could do. But every drug has both beneficial effects and not-so-beneficial side effects. Whenever you purposely change the way your body works, it affects other things in some way. This means many seventy-year-olds take many medications with no certainty about how they interact. My grandparents lived into their eighties and nineties with no medications. It's not that humans have changed. Instead, culture has redefined normal as taking medication for every little thing. So, if I don't want be on all kinds of medications in twenty to thirty years, I need to take care of myself today.

Let's look back at society's normal—overweight, low energy, and overly medicated as they age. No thank you. We don't have to accept this, but to avoid it, we must reject society's definition of normal.

BIG IDEAS

Normal does not necessarily mean healthy.

You can and should reject society's definition of normal as your normal.

Our goal is healthy, not perfect.

ACTION STEPS

Go to the mall or another public place and simply watch
people for ten to fifteen minutes. Without criticism,
take an honest assessment: Do people look healthy?
Do they have a healthy bodyweight?

Go back to your dream:
Where do you want to be in one year? In ten years?

Write a list of "normal" physical things in our culture
that you don't want any part of.

PUT THAT MACHINE TO WORK

Our body is a machine for living. –LEO TOLSTOY[16]

A few years back, I needed a car because mine had well over two hundred thousand miles and needed repairs that far exceeded its value. I was given an old Honda Accord stick shift that had been sitting for several years. They told me it was in good running condition. I sold my beat-up old car and went to get the Honda. It was a cold day, and I quickly learned that the heater was broken as I shivered violently driving home. My unease continued to grow when I realized I could only go about forty miles per hour on the highway; it wouldn't accelerate any faster. Then reality hit me: this is my car and the only one I have or will have for some time. Regret kicked in. This car had once been a good car but had been neglected. Its performance was now terrible.

So I filled the gas tank with super, even though it only needed regular. Then I got the oil changed and the heater fixed. Next, I took it on a long drive to completely burn out the old gas. By this time, it was up to fifty miles per hour, which continued to increase over time. As I continued to use the highest-octane gas, the engine cleaned out, and I drove that car for another two hundred and fifty thousand miles. It was a great machine but needed to be cared for and utilized in the right way.

I NEGLECTED MY BODY

My body is a great machine, but I neglected it. In the same way I needed to clean out and take care of that car, my body needed the same treatment. My body didn't need higher octane gas, but it needed highly nutritional foods to both clean it out and build it up. It needed to rebuild muscle and increase the strength and efficiency of my heart and lungs. Just as I celebrated every time that Honda went five miles per hour faster, I celebrated every time I added five minutes on the elliptical or could add a few pounds to the barbell or machine.

LEARNING HOW THE MACHINE WORKS

I became fascinated as a teen with how the human body works. As a young athlete, my passion drove me to learn how it functioned. My body was my vessel to win. Any success was due more to passion than ability. As an athlete, I had average skill but tried to outwork everyone to win. Freshman year I began playing football at 5' 4" and 115 pounds. I spent the next eight years of my life building up to six feet and 226 pounds, almost always competing against bigger, faster, stronger people, so the weight room became my home and *Muscle & Fitness* magazine my educator.

I began college as a special education major but tore my ACL in my left knee and had major surgery my sophomore year. I spent four to six hours a day in the training room every day rehabbing that knee. I was hooked. I wanted to be an athletic trainer, which meant switching my major to physical education so I could specialize in athletic training. I followed that with studying applied physiology and nutrition in graduate school at Columbia University and doing a summer internship with the Kansas City Chiefs. I spent over a decade in my teens and twenties totally focused on learning everything I could about the body and putting it into practice in my personal life. Here are a few lessons I learned.

THE BODY IS A MACHINE

The body works in predictable—almost mechanical—ways by design. The body is hardwired to breathe, pump blood, and digest food without any thought or action. It is a biochemical machine that releases hormones and enzymes to keep balance and cause actions to take place. The body's first goal is survival, so it constantly works to maintain a sense of stability and health called homeostasis.

> **Homeostasis:** the tendency of a system, especially the physiological system of higher animals, to maintain internal stability, owing to the coordinated response of its parts to any situation or stimulus that would tend to disturb its normal condition or function.[17]

To maintain optimal health, our body signals what it needs. If we are dehydrated (have insufficient water in our body), hormones that signal thirst are produced. When our blood sugar is low and we are not burning fat for energy, our body releases other hormones that cause hunger so that we'll eat. Every hormone is counterbalanced by another to signal, in case we drink too much water or eat too much food. I studied these physiological functions for over a decade with the goal of achieving optimal physical performance.

THE BODY ADAPTS

How the body adapts to the stress we put on it forms the foundation for both optimal athletic performance and physical health. We can place stress (exercise) on our body that essentially forces the body to build stronger muscles and burn fat as energy. We can eat certain foods at certain times that cause the body to function more efficiently, build muscle, and choose to burn fat.

THE BODY DOESN'T THINK; IT REACTS

Since the body is a machine, it simply functions. It's more complicated than a car, but let's compare. If we fill a gas tank with fifteen gallons of gas and get twenty-five miles per gallon, we can drive three hundred miles and still have some gas in the tank. If we change the oil, it lubricates the engine for the next three to five thousand miles. Over time different parts like brakes, tires, and filters need to be routinely replaced. In our body, food is our gas, water is our oil, and nutrients replace our skin, bones, muscles, hair etc. over time. If we use cheap gas, don't change the oil and other fluids, and don't replace the worn-out parts, the car will break down sooner than if we do those maintenance chores. Same with the body. When we put in the best nutrients and sufficient water, it functions better and lasts longer. How we eat and exercise has tremendous influence on how the body will respond.

PLAN YOUR SUCCESS

After you have a clear dream and vision, you must create and execute a plan. Otherwise, your dream is only a wish. Creating a plan requires knowledge and organization; know your subject and then make a systematic plan for improvement.

First, know how your body works. Understand the relationship between extra fat and decreased energy. Memorize the process of shedding excess weight. Then, apply the basics over time. It's like making a deposit in the bank every week; whether you add a little money or a lot, it will add up over time if you contribute weekly. If you want to build your account faster, add more each week. Same with fat loss but in reverse. If you subtract fat weekly, it will go away; if you want to lose it faster, just increase the rate of loss. To keep it off, it has to be done the right way.

What am I supposed to focus on? So glad you asked. Remember our three main goals:

1. **Build muscle:** Muscle is your calorie-burning engine.
2. **Burn fat:** Your goal is not to lose weight but to burn fat.
3. **Eat right:** Eat the right foods at the right time.

If you do these three things, you will be stronger, have less fat, and have more daily energy. Sign me up! Done the right way, you will also come out with a much faster metabolism, which will allow you to stay leaner for *the rest of your life.*

Everybody wants these results, but few get them, and even fewer people keep them. Be different; be better. Remember, you can do this because behavior is more important than knowledge, and you are in charge of your behavior, your choices. You must transform the knowledge into action on a daily basis.

Your body is a magnificent machine that responds in certain ways to certain actions. It's time for you to take control and do the right things that will make your body do what you want it to. You can do this!

THE BODY GROWS IN ENDURANCE AND STRENGTH WHEN STRESSED

Let's go back to our three goals and revisit how they help us maximize our muscle development, decrease our fat levels, and increase our daily energy.

1. **Build muscle:** Muscle is your fat-burning tool; the more muscle you have, the more you burn calories and fat.

2. **Burn fat:** We must target and purposely burn fat rather than aiming to just lose weight.

3. **Eat right:** Eating the right foods at the right times supplies our body with nutrients to build muscle, increase overall health, and direct the body to burn unwanted fat.

Here are some basic definitions in layman's terms that we will dig into in greater detail:

Metabolism: the rate your body burns calories
Hypertrophy: muscle growth caused by resistance training
Endurance: the ability to perform aerobic exercise for extended periods
Fat Burning: targeting fat as your source of energy during exercise and afterwards

YOUR BODY IS A MACHINE; IT DOESN'T HAVE FEELINGS

Your physical body doesn't care what you eat or what you do. On some level, it is a machine (organism) that simply responds to what you do. Lift heavier weights three times a week for a year, and guess what? You will add muscle over time. Get on the elliptical every day for a month for thirty minutes and improve your diet, and you will lose fat. Eat regular, healthy meals and snacks at the right times, and your metabolism will speed up and you'll store less fat.

This may seem too simple for some. But simple things done consistently over time will cause your body to react in extremely predictable ways. Your body doesn't think, reason, or feel; it only responds to what you choose to do. Use this fact to build confidence that your efforts and choices will get results.

BIG IDEAS

Your body is a machine that functions according to principles.

Your body adapts in predictable ways to the stress (exercise) you put on it.

You have a great deal of control over your body.

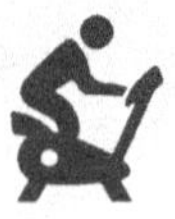

ACTION STEPS

Learn about how your body works by reading, watching videos, etc.

Create plans on how to increase your exercise levels.

Commit to consistency over time.

TRAIN YOUR METABOLISM

METABOLISM

Biology, Physiology: the sum of the physical and chemical process in an organism by which its material substance is produced, maintained, and destroyed, and by which energy is made available.[18]

Whenever I've needed to burn fat over the years, I've had one goal: build my metabolism. Notice, I didn't say "lose weight" or "diet." Remember, your metabolism is the rate your body burns calories. I knew that with diligence in eating right and increasing cardio and weightlifting, I would hit a point where my metabolism kicked into a higher gear. Weight would then come off. Increased metabolism is also key to maintaining desired weight in the long term.

I am convinced that training your metabolism is the most important thing you can do to lose fat and keep it off. Fat consists of extra calories that we ate but did not burn off. To burn fat, we must burn more calories than we eat. (Remember: It's not rocket science.) When we burn more calories than we eat day after day, the body breaks down the extra fat as it is used for energy. It's simple math, people.

FASTER METABOLISM = MORE CALORIES BURNED

You know the skinny guy who can eat anything and never gain a pound? His metabolism is super-fast. Natural metabolism is greatly determined by genetics, but the good news is we have the ability to speed it up or slow it down based on our exercise and eating patterns.

If we speed it up, we burn more calories when we are sitting down, moving around, and even sleeping. We can better understand our metabolism by comparing it to an engine. If you have two cars taking the same trip, but one is a four-cylinder engine and the other is an eight-cylinder engine, the eight-cylinder engine uses more gas. It's simple: more cylinders (bigger engine or, in our case, more muscle) require more fuel to make them go. With increased cardiovascular exercise, you will also increase fat-burning enzymes within your body, which is like increasing an engine's revolutions per minute.

Imagine two cars sitting next to each other in park, but one guy keeps his foot on the gas, which increases the engine's revolutions per minute and burns more gas just sitting there. Increasing your metabolism is like increasing the number of cylinders in your engine and your revolutions per minute. If we can increase our metabolism, we will burn more energy on a daily basis, which adds up over time.

THREE BASIC STEPS TO INCREASING METABOLISM

I: Eat Frequently and at the Right Time

Our bodies are designed to survive. After air and water, the most important thing we need is food. Food supplies the energy we need to both survive and thrive. If food is scarce, for any reason, we eat less frequently. Our bodies adjust by slowing our metabolism down to conserve energy.

Our ancestors benefitted from this system; during crop failure or times of drought, their bodies knew how to compensate for fewer available calories. In times when food supply was low, our ancestors ate only one or two meals a day until the harvest came in or the fruits ripened or animals or fish were available, so the body slowed down and used fewer calories.

In modern times, we essentially have an unlimited supply of food in America. If you try to restrict, to eat only one meal a day to lose weight, you are signaling to your body that there is a crisis, a famine. You are essentially forcing your body to slow its metabolism to help you survive the lack.

Thermogenic Effect

This principle states that each time a person eats, their metabolism speeds up as they digest the food. One example is a study reported by the *American Journal of Clinical Nutrition*. In the study, ten women who ate regularly scheduled meals lost weight while eating the same food at irregular times led to weight gain and reduced insulin sensitivity.[19] One of the healthy trends of recent weight-loss efforts has been a more focused effort to eat well and increase exercise, which is a much healthier approach than the past several decades, which often had a thin-at-any-cost approach.

Dieting Has Changed

In decades past, one of the main strategies of losing weight was skipping breakfast and lunch and then eating a big dinner. Exercise and food choice were often neglected or not part of the program. A dieter's metabolism would be trained to slow down for twenty-four hours due to lack of food and then taught to store fat and nutrients from the one big meal. Many people rapidly lost weight following this pattern, but when they returned to a regular eating schedule, they did so with a slower metabolism, which had been trained to store calories by adapting to the once-a-day eating routine. Luckily, this type of mass thinking has been replaced by a healthier eating and exercise model.

On the other hand, each time we eat, our metabolism speeds up. When we eat three regular meals a day and healthy snacks, it signals to our body that it will get food regularly—no famine in sight—and can keep burning calories at a normal rate. Total calorie intake still impacts weight gain/loss, but eating on a regular schedule has been shown to be a factor in healthier weight loss.

One of the greatest lessons from my forty-pound fat loss was the importance of timing for meals and snacks. I stopped eating after eight at night. Near the end, I did not start eating until noon. I always ate three meals between noon and eight o'clock but learned that by not eating late and delaying my first meal until noon, I increased my body's fat burning. Generally, I always eat breakfast, which works well for losing weight slowly and consistently or maintaining. The timing of meals can make a big difference; I found it helpful on a short-term basis.

2: Increase Cardiovascular Exercise or HIIT

Cardiovascular or aerobic exercise breaks down fat to supply the energy needed to do the exercise. Aerobic exercise can be defined simply as repetitive exercise using large muscle groups that increases oxygen intake for an extended period of time. These exercises include walking, jogging, hiking, swimming, Stairmaster™, elliptical, rowing and varied aerobics classes for at least 12 minutes but generally 20 minutes or longer.

In our engine story, increased metabolism is like increasing the revolutions per minute of an engine. There are times when an engine's timing is off and the revolutions per minute are too high. This means the engine is working harder than it should and will burn gas, which is a bad thing. But when we talk about our bodies, we want our internal engine working faster and burning more fat. One cardiovascular session can speed up your metabolism for the next twelve to twenty-four hours. The greater the intensity and duration of the exercise session, the greater the effect of extended fat burning post exercise.[20] This means you not only burn more calories from the exercise itself but will continue to burn increased calories for at least the next twelve hours, which adds up over time.

3: Build Muscle

I drive a lot, so I purposely buy four-cylinder cars. They have enough power to go eighty miles per hour and enough pickup to speed up when needed. That's all I need. I don't want a six cylinder because it would use too much gas. Never mind an eight cylinder; I would go broke.

But when it comes to my body, I want more cylinders to burn more calories. This means more muscle, which is active, calorie-burning tissue. Muscle burns calories when you sit, move, and even sleep. Simply put, the more muscle you have, the more calories you will burn each day.

Resistance Training

To build muscle, you must stress the muscles with added resistance. This includes lifting weights, machines, kettlebells, and bodyweight exercises like push-ups, pull-ups, planks, and HIIT training. When you stress muscles, they adapt by growing stronger and larger; therefore, they burn more calories. Consistent resistance sessions over time produce consistent growth. The general rule is to stress the muscles, give them a day to rest, and then get after it again. This may mean working out total body three days a week, or if people want to do resistance training more often, they may work half the body one day and rotate to the other muscle groups the next day. This would allow a person to do resistance training six days a week but have a full day of rest between working the same muscles. As I ramped up my weight-loss efforts, this was the pattern I used, going from three days a week of resistance to six days a week but alternating muscle groups. More detail on this later.

I DON'T WANT TO GET TOO BIG

I often hear, "I don't want to get too big," when I talk to people about lifting weights or using other forms of resistance training. In thirty-five years of going to gyms and in working with athletes, students, and all types of people, I have never seen someone look in the mirror and proclaim, "My muscles are just too big!" Male, female, young, old—I've never heard it.

This fear is a myth. People don't understand how much time is required and how difficult it is to build truly large muscles. It takes years to build a significant amount of increased muscle, and it disappears pretty quickly if you stop working out.

If people feel they are too big, it's likely an issue of having more fat than they want, not too much muscle. For women, adding muscle accentuates curves and tones up the body; it doesn't create a bulky, masculine physique. Women don't have testosterone to the degree men do, so they can't build large, bulky muscles like men. Yes, they can build muscle and be fit, but a different biochemistry and hormonal system means a different result for women. That being said, women do benefit greatly from resistance training.

Bottom line: if you build your metabolism, it is the healthiest and most effective way for short- and long-term weight loss and maintenance. The more we plan our workouts and food choices, the faster and greater we can speed up our metabolism. Let's start to take a detailed look at achieving our three main goals.

BIG IDEAS

Metabolism is the rate your body burns calories.

To increase your metabolism, do these three things:

a. Eat frequent, sufficient meals at the right times.

b. Burn fat through cardiovascular exercise or HIIT.

c. Build muscle through resistance training.

You can train your body to burn fat, not just calories.

ACTION STEPS

Time meals and snacks and pay attention to food content.

Plan your workouts to include cardio (and other fat-burning exercises) and resistance training to build muscle.

Be consistent. Burning fat and building muscle are two different processes that both take time.

BUILD MUSCLE

Whatever muscles I have are the product of my own hard work and nothing else. –Evelyn Ashford[21]

I knew reaching my goal meant building maximum muscle. More muscle burns more calories and allows increased workout intensity. A mental shift also takes place through both physical improvements and a sense of ongoing accomplishment. Both act as powerful motivators to keep going and to keep going harder over time. Building muscle can also be done by anyone who puts in the work.

Evelyn Ashford won the 1984 Olympic gold medal in the hundred meters, establishing her as the fastest female in the world at this event. Her quote declares that her muscle development came from work, not a genetic gift. Compared to you and me, she was probably more gifted, but amongst her peers, she saw her success as the result of hard work, not lineage or luck. This confirms the idea that anyone can build muscle if they put in the work.

INCREASED MUSCLE IS FOUNDATIONAL TO A BETTER METABOLISM

Muscle is active, healthy, calorie-burning tissue. The more you have, the more calories you burn when you sit, stand, sleep, or exercise. Muscle makes men more masculine and women curvier and toned. Increased muscle makes all people feel stronger and decreases aches, pains, and injuries—all leading to increased confidence.

You build muscle by gradually increasing the resistance you place on muscles. This is most commonly achieved through free weights (barbells and dumbbells) and weight machines, but kettlebells and body weight exercises, like traditional calisthenics (push-ups, pull-ups, sit-ups, and crunches), and newer exercises and programs, like HIIT, are also effective.

ANYONE CAN BUILD MORE MUSCLE

Anyone can build more muscle. That's a pretty confidant statement, right? I can say this because of a biological principle. When you stress muscles in a controlled manner that gradually increases the stress you put on them, they will positively adapt by improved nervous system response and increased functional strength, thereby building larger, stronger muscle fibers.

OVERLOAD PRINCIPLE: YOUR KEY TO PROGRESSIVE IMPROVEMENT

Overload Principle: Fundamental theory of training in which exercise at an intensity above that normally attained will induce highly specific adaptations, enabling the body to function more efficiently. Overload is applied to manipulating combinations of training frequency, intensity, and duration.[22]

Overload is the key principle of physical progression. Whatever exercise routine you start, you want to begin at a level that will not produce excessive soreness or injury and then gradually build up over time. You might do two sets of eight repetitions with forty pounds on a bench press machine. Over time, it becomes two sets of ten repetitions, then two sets of twelve repetitions, and then you add ten pounds and start again with two sets of eight repetitions with fifty pounds. Fast-forward a couple of months and you may be doing two sets of eight repetitions with eighty pounds. The gradual overload will cause the body to build larger, stronger muscle fibers able to lift increasing amounts of weight, with the last several repetitions being close to maximal effort while maintaining proper form. This causes muscular growth: "hypertrophy" in technical terms.

Hypertrophy: Increase in volume of a tissue or organ produced entirely by enlargement of existing cells.[23]

The consistent application of the overload principle causes existing muscle fibers to grow in both size and strength. Generally, these changes are not visible at first but, over time, can become physically apparent in muscle tone, body contour, and shape, followed by clearly visible muscular growth.

MAINTAINING AND BUILDING MUSCLE

It may sound funny, but maintaining your current muscle mass is a process. Remember, do nothing, and your body will adapt to no stress by allowing muscles to deteriorate. The technical word for this is *atrophy*.

Atrophy: A wasting away of the body or of an organ or part, as from defective nutrition or nerve damage; degeneration, decline, or decrease, as from disuse.[24]

An example of atrophy is the man who had a strong chest and muscular arms as a teen and young adult but now has thinner arms and chest and a slumped-over back. All you have to do is nothing, which will result in muscular deterioration.

We've all had the experience of lifting something that once was easily lifted and now it's not so easy or, even worse, now lifting it causes us to pull a muscle. What to do? Hit the gym and put that overload principle to work. Start where you are and slowly increase your reps or the intensity and frequency of your muscle-building workouts.

REPETITION, INTENSITY, AND FREQUENCY

One of the ways to break plateaus or reach new goals is to amplify a few factors in your workout:

Repetitions (reps): The number of times a weight is lifted, or an exercise is executed. You increase results when you add reps (i.e., moving from ten pushups to fifteen or two sets of eight to two sets of twelve).

Intensity: Increase intensity by adding repetitions, increasing resistance, or taking a shorter rest between sets.

Frequency: The number of overall workouts is the frequency. For example, I went from lifting entire body one or two days a week to three; then I alternated body parts but lifted six days a week. (Monday/Wednesday/Friday, I did chest/legs/abs, and Tuesday/Thursday/Saturday were for back/shoulders/arms.)

RPE: RATED PERCEIVED EXERTION SCALE

We can also measure intensity through the concept of rated perceived exertion (RPE), a concept where a person gauges their effort on the level of exertion they are putting out. Following is a scale to illustrate:

0 = no effort

3 = light

5 = medium

7 = heavy

9 = very heavy

10 = maximum effort

When it comes to muscle building, all repetitions are not equal in creating overload. For an untrained person, doing two sets of eight with forty pounds on a bench press machine may be an RPE of nine. After a week or two, it may be an RPE of five. Because his muscles got stronger, the same weight and reps became easier. The pattern of adding reps would continue until you could do twelve. Add weight and then reps over time to up the RPE and repeat.

This is subjective, depending on a person's perception and physical condition. To build muscle, you should keep in the RPE range of five to nine and the repetition range of eight to twelve reps per exercise. If I am able to do three sets of twelve reps with one hundred pounds on the bench press machine, but am only doing two sets of ten at eighty pounds, my RPE is probably only around four or so—insufficient to create overload and muscle growth.

SLOW AND STEADY IS THE GOAL

Your body takes time to build larger and stronger muscle fibers. This is why you must eat well. You simply will not build muscle if you don't have enough protein or have a drastic calorie deficit.

Do too much too soon and you will cause excessive muscular pain or injury to tendons and joints. You can apply this to any exercise. One of your goals is increase endurance by adding distance or time to an exercise. You hope to cause the body to adapt to the overload you put on it. I went from doing the elliptical for twelve minutes to sixty minutes over time. This allowed my heart, lungs, and leg muscles time to adapt to the gradually increasing overload.

In terms of building stronger muscles and increasing endurance, the overload principle is your new best friend.

EVERY INCREASE IS PROGRESS

Be patient and be steady. You are building a better body through science/physiology. If you have the attitude that every time you hit the gym you will do more reps or more weight in different exercises, this will keep you motivated and force your body to grow stronger muscles. This won't happen every day with every exercise, but all should trend upwards over time.

Muscle then becomes your calorie/fat burner, which will help you reach *and* maintain your goal weight once achieved. Simple, steady overload over time is the key to muscle-building progress. Your body adapts to the stress put on it. Every time you push your muscles slightly harder than before—and then eat right and rest—your muscles will grow stronger. Remember, it's science.

EYE OF THE TIGER

We keep the eye of the tiger (remember attitude is *huge*) by continually challenging ourselves with the overload principle and pushing ourselves based on RPE. If I did dumbbell curls with twenty pounds, then my goal is to bump up to twenty-five pounds. If I was only able to do a plank for twenty seconds, then my next goal would be to hold it twenty-five to thirty seconds. Constantly challenge yourself to lift a little more, go a little longer, or add an additional exercise that used to be too difficult.

Simply put, you lose the eye of the tiger when you get comfortable or when you stop chasing your next challenge. Progress also feeds passion. Every time you can do something that you couldn't do a day, week, or month ago, it motivates you. You want to turn your workouts into motivational challenges where you push yourself to get better every time. This will build positive momentum to fuel your ongoing efforts. Eye of the tiger, baby!

FOCUS ON FULL-BODY OR MULTIPLE-MUSCLE EXERCISES

A good principle to build muscle is to use full-body or multiple muscle exercises over isolation exercises. Here's a list of exercises and the muscle groups targeted:

- Bench Press: chest, shoulders, and triceps
- Upright Rows: shoulders, trapezius, and biceps
- Squats: quadriceps (front of thigh), lower back, hamstring (back of thigh)
- Deadlifts: lower back, quadriceps, hamstring, and trapezius
- Kettlebell Swings

By using full-body or multiple-muscle movements, you incorporate large, multiple muscle groups, causing greater overall muscle development and strength. These tend also to build greater functional strength in sports or everyday life.

Machines and isolated exercises also have benefits of stressing individual muscles and can be used when other body parts are injured. In fact, let's talk about avoiding injury.

AVOIDING EXTREME PAIN

No pain, no gain . . . uhhhh, maybe? –Jack Redmond

I'm not saying working out will never be uncomfortable, but one of the reasons people's weight loss doesn't last is because they choose a painful path. Many lose weight, but if you check back in a year or two, they gained it back and then some. One reason it doesn't last is because they embraced a painful lifestyle that helped them effectively lose weight, but it was too painful to maintain long term or caused physical damage that led to not working out. Setbacks can result from experiencing pain during workouts or from actual injury by trying a level of intensity the body isn't ready for.

PAIN VS. DISCOMFORT

If working out is new to you or if you have been inactive for a while, you will experience muscle soreness. In fact, if you never feel any discomfort during or the day after exercise, your workouts may not be challenging enough. Slight discomfort during and after exercise can be fine, but pain during or after is a signal that you are either working out too hard or progressing in intensity too quickly.

MUSCLE SORENESS VS. MUSCLE OR JOINT PAIN

Differentiating soreness from pain may seem confusing, so let me describe and simplify. Delayed onset muscle soreness (DOMS) is the normal, low-level pain a person experiences when starting a more strenuous exercise program. Slight soreness in the muscle itself can be fine, especially when you are new to the exercise. This type of mild pain may increase for two to three days and then start to fade.

Extreme pain, however, is telling you that you went too hard, too soon. Over time, your muscles will adapt, so pain should not be ongoing. If you are experiencing pain in your joints and tendons, that is a signal you are overdoing it. This can also indicate you are moving toward or have caused injury, especially if you are feeling sharp or chronic pain. This will require medical attention if it doesn't resolve itself with basic rest and ice in forty-eight to seventy-two hours.

TOO MUCH TOO SOON

If I got a dollar for everyone I knew who did too much too soon, I would be rich. Remember, our goal is gradual and sustainable lifestyle and lifetime change. For instance, I've had many friends who've never worked out consistently join a CrossFit® gym. They go from being a couch potato to doing explosive, extreme exercises. Within the first week, their knee tendons and shoulder tendons hurt. Pain means swelling and some level of tissue damage. CrossFit and other high-intensity programs can be highly beneficial but require a certain level of fitness and proper recuperation time. One of my friends recently told me all his friends told him to "work through the pain." So, he kept going, exacerbating the joint pain so much that he stopped working out. Last time I checked, he had gained weight. I'm not against a mild level of discomfort, but pain is a signal you are doing too much too soon.

YES, YOU NEED TO WORK HARD AND SACRIFICE

To reach your goal, you must work. You will experience discomfort and be challenged to live differently. If you have a real goal, it will not be easy. Be steady, be healthy, but also be smart. You can do it, but to sustain it, you must do it right. Consistently apply the overload principle, and over time, you will build muscle.

BIG IDEAS

Increased muscle will cause faster metabolism.

Gradual, consistent increases in stress on muscles
will cause them to grow stronger and
larger (hypertrophy) over time.

Overload occurs when we increase the reps, intensity,
or frequency of resistance training.

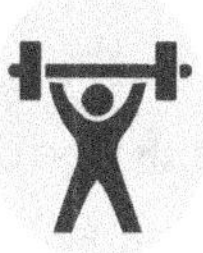

ACTION STEPS

Perform resistance training two to three days per week on each muscle group.

Consistently challenge yourself to increase reps, intensity, or frequency in some exercise every time you work out.

Attempt to keep your RPE between five to nine in a range of eight to twelve reps in each resistance exercise.

Here is a short review on resistance training principles and sample exercises and routines:

Please consult a physician any time you begin an exercise routine or have any limitations or pre-existing conditions that need to be considered as you create a workout plan.

Overload Principle – gradually increase stress on muscles by adding repetitions or weight to each exercise. This can be applied to any form of exercise.

1. Gradually increase reps from 8 to 12 per set
2. Add 5 – 10 lbs. to exercise and go back to sets of 8 repetition.

Weightlifting Principles:

1. Do at least 3 sets per major muscle group.
2. Do resistance training 2-3 times per week with 1-2 days of rest between exercising the same muscles.
3. Focus on large muscle groups first – i.e. chest, back, legs then shoulders, arms, abs.

Key Exercises

Chest – bench press, incline press, dips

Back – pull downs, seated rows, 1 arm rows

Legs – squats, leg press, leg extensions (quadriceps),

leg curls (hamstrings)

Shoulders – shoulder press, upright rows, lateral raises

Triceps – triceps pushdowns, triceps extensions (ez curl bar)

Biceps – barbell curl, dumbbell curls

Abs – crunches, hanging leg raises, planks

Kettle Bell Routine

– Start with 1 set of 10 of each and progress to 3 sets per exercise

- Kettlebell Swings 2 arm
- 1 arm lunges – holding kb overhead, alternate legs
- KB thrusters – squat to shoulder press movement
- KB – 1 arm snatches – right and left
- KB squats
- KB deadlift

You can do these and other exercises as a routine with 10-30 second rest between.

I also like the Tabata® method meaning 20 seconds of exercise followed by 10 seconds rest before moving to next exercise.

HIIT Training – designed to burn fat and build muscle

These are bodyweight exercises that include traditional calisthenics and other exercises:

- Jumping jacks
- Push ups
- Squats
- Inch worms
- Burpees (can modify for different intensities/abilities)
- High knees
- Planks (multiple variations)
- Flutterkick squats
- Woodchop – hands to knees
- Standing criss cross crunch
- Mountain climbers

There are many online workouts to get you started and progress in intensity over time for each of these forms of resistance training.

CHAPTER 9

BURN FAT

Dear fat,
Prepare to die…
XOXO, Me

To reach my goal weight, I had to target fat burning because burning calories differs from purposely targeting fat. Yes, you will burn fat over time if you simply use more calories than you eat; this is foundational. But the greater the focus and effort to target fat, the quicker you can purposely burn and get rid of unwanted fat.

BUILDING A FAT-BURNING METABOLISM

The faster your metabolism, we now know, the easier it is to burn fat and keep it off. We've also learned that a faster metabolism burns more calories when you are sitting, standing, exercising, and even sleeping. We need to get that engine going! How do we do that? You guessed it: build muscle, burn fat, and eat the right foods at the right times.

This is our familiar drumbeat. Learn the beat; live the beat. Losing fat is simple. It's not easy for everyone, but over time, if you learn basic principles and consistently do them, they will work.

Many will ask, "If this is so simple, why are so many people carrying around unwanted, unhealthy fat?" Remember, it's about behavior more than knowledge of principles. Our world is full of people who know better but don't do what they know. Everyone knows running up credit cards is bad, yet many people are in debt.

Growing up, I never understood how people could smoke cigarettes when the label on the side of the box literally tells you that they will give you cancer. See? The knowledge is there, but we still have the freedom to choose the wrong behavior. We first have to know the right thing, but then we must go on to win the battle of the mind and consistently choose the right thing.

BUT I DON'T KNOW HOW TO DO THIS

Well, you probably do. If not, I will teach you, or at least I will add to what you already know. But, as you have heard me say before, this is not rocket science. Consider three simple approaches to losing fat. Which approach most resonates with you?

1. **It's science:** The body works a certain way. When you eat and exercise certain ways, the body will respond accordingly. Brilliant, right? That's what I learned doing three master's degrees at Ivy League Columbia University. Physiological processes are set and can be depended on. Your body will follow these principles or rules.

2. **It's math:** If you burn more calories than you eat, you will lose

weight; it's straight-up Cro-Magnon logic. If you can figure out how to pick things up and put things down, you can do this. If you burn more calories than you eat every day, you will lose weight. The smarter you do it, the faster it will go and the longer it will stay off.

3. **It's an art:** How does this all work with your body and what you like to do and eat? You have to take the basic principles and finesse them to work in your life. Weight loss can be a little more complicated based on your physiology, hormonal stages, metabolism, and possible physical limitations, but you can and will make progress if you are committed to doing so. Yes, the principles are universal but will work a little differently in different people or either in the same person at different ages, based on changing life circumstances.

MY BEST FRIEND: THE ELLIPTICAL MACHINE

The one exercise I can point to as the most beneficial in my weight loss is the elliptical machine. If you are unfamiliar with this machine, it works both arms and legs simultaneously. Your legs travel in an arc, similar to a cross-country skiing motion, with your arms pushing and pulling levers. The movement is somewhere between jogging and cross-country skiing. I knew if I got on the elliptical and kept going, I would burn fat. Consistent effort for an extended period of time at the right intensity burns fat.

Success means having the courage, the determination, and the will to become the person you believe you were meant to be. –Darren Hardy Quotes[25]

THIRTY MINUTES A DAY ON THE ELLIPTICAL

One of my goals in reaching 190 was that from January 1, 2020, to February 20, 2020, I would spend at least thirty minutes every day on the elliptical. For the first week and a half, I did not enjoy this daily effort. I felt tired. It felt like work, and I had zero excitement about it. I had been doing about twenty minutes each time I went to the gym, but I bumped that up to seven days a week and thirty minutes each time. Around day ten or eleven, I was on the elliptical and was not feeling it. But when I pushed through, something changed physically and psychologically. I felt an energy burst and a mental change that I hadn't felt in years. Then the light bulb went on: I could have felt better every single day for the last ten years if I'd started these changes sooner.

I needed this breakthrough, especially since I had been working out to lesser degrees for a couple years and not feeling any great benefit. Increased intensity and frequency helped me see my past efforts were somewhat beneficial but ultimately insufficient.

HIIT EXERCISE AND FAT BURNING DURING AND POST EXERCISE

While on my fat-loss journey, two friends who do personal training for a living kept pushing me to do HIIT workouts. Unfortunately, due to my spine injury, I couldn't do them. HIIT is popular because these workouts use bodyweight, so they can be done anywhere with no equipment in a short amount of time with great results. Let's look at the benefits.

High intensity interval training (HIIT) workouts are ten to thirty minutes of intense exercise designed to increase heart rate, burn calories, and build muscle. One study comparing thirty minutes of HIIT exercise to steady-state aerobics on stationary bike or treadmill (at 70 percent maximum heart rate) and lifting weights demonstrated a 25-30 percent higher caloric expenditure in HIIT versus the other three exercise routines.[26]

Studies also show that HIIT routines lead to greater fat-burning resting energy expenditure (REE) post exercise in women[27] and the same twenty-four hour respiratory exchange ratio (RER) for HIIT and traditional cardiovascular exercise, even though HIIT is performed for less time.[28] Another study showed how sprint interval exercise, similar to HIIT, showed increased oxygen intake and fat oxidation (fat burning) in men.[29]

HIIT has been shown to increase caloric burn during exercise and provide tremendous post-exercise fat-burning capacity. These exercises are also attractive because the benefits can be realized in shorter workout times while utilizing body weight exercises that can be performed anywhere at no cost. HIIT burns fat by putting the body in the target heart range to burn fat for the duration of the workout.

FAT BREAKDOWN

Fat breakdown is a simple chemical process that requires oxygen to be added to the fat molecule during exercise to break down fat into carbon dioxide and water.

$$O_2 + C_{58}H_{12}O_6 \rightarrow CO_2 + H_2O + \text{energy}$$

If you look at the fat molecule of $C_{58}H_{12}O_6$, you can see that it has fifty-eight carbons, twelve hydrogens, and only six oxygen molecules. You must add O_2 to the fat to get the right ratios of CO_2 and H_2O. At some point, it's just math. You have a lot of carbons, so you need a lot of oxygen to make CO_2 and H_2O.

During cardiovascular exercise, increased breathing takes in the needed extra oxygen, and the body demands energy production to continue the exercise. Three basic things then take place: the body breathes out the excess CO_2 and the H_2O is used by the body as sweat; and increased vapor in breath and rest is absorbed and used by the body; and energy given off by the chemical breakdown of fat supplies the energy needed for the exercise.

TIME FACTOR

The amount of time we spend doing cardiovascular exercise affects the amount of fat burned. Like a car, the longer you drive, the more gas you use. The longer you do cardio, the more fat you burn. It's simple math, but it gets better. The longer you go affects the amount of fat that gets burned as increased enzymes and other metabolic factors increase the fat-burning process, like a campfire that burns stronger over time.

PERCENTAGE OF FAT BURNED

You have to do at least twelve minutes of cardio to get into a significant fat-burning zone. When you first start exercise, you are predominately burning carbohydrates. This is good as you are burning calories, but you are not breaking down fat.

Let's take a look at a walk or jog. When you start, you may be burning 90 percent carbohydrate and 10 percent fat. At six minutes, it may be 70 percent carbohydrate and 30 percent fat. After twelve minutes, it may shift to 45 percent carbohydrate and 55 percent fat. At twenty minutes, it may be 40 percent carbohydrate and 60 percent fat. I am not saying this is an exact scientific fact in terms of percentages, but I am using it as an illustration of the principle. These numbers would differ from person to person and depend greatly on their state of conditioning and training.

FAT-BURNING ENZYMES

When I do seminars on weight loss, I show pictures of two men. The first is a large overweight man who is easily over three hundred pounds. Then I show a picture of a lean Kenyan marathon runner and ask the question: "If both men start jogging, which person burns a higher percentage of fat?" I get many confused faces as people are trying to figure out if I am trying to trick them. For most, the gut feeling is the big guy. He has more fat, so he must use more fat is the logic. The answer is the opposite. The extremely thin, conditioned athlete has trained his body to use fat as an energy source, while the larger, unconditioned man will rely on carbohydrates as his energy source.

THAT'S NOT FAIR

You are correct, but in the real world, fair often doesn't matter. It's not fair, but it is physiology. It's science, so it doesn't matter what we think. However, we can use knowledge to our benefit. Since fat produces more sustainable energy, it is the body's preferred source of energy during extended physical effort. The Kenyan marathoner has trained his body to use fat instead of carbohydrate. Ready for another unfair reality? The overweight man burns mostly carbohydrate because he gets tired and stops exercising before his body switches over to burning predominately fat. This means his workout was likely unpleasant, possibly painful, and probably ineffective in burning any fat.

WALKING KEEPS YOU IN THE FAT-BURNING RANGE

By walking, you are increasing the need to produce energy and taking in additional oxygen for this chemical reaction to take place. Different intensities of exercise utilize different energy systems in the body. The reason you can't sprint for two miles is because you can't take in sufficient oxygen to burn fat; instead you burn carbohydrates, which offer less total energy than fat. So, the lower intensity of walking allows your body to choose to specifically break down fat. Any exercise will burn a combination of fat and carbohydrate, but walking targets fat breakdown.

HOW CAN I KNOW MY FAT-BURNING RANGE?

One of the greatest lessons I learned in my forty-pound weight loss was to focus on burning fat instead of just burning calories. One of the keys is to exercise with your heart beating in a range that will target fat. It's simple. If your heart is beating too fast and you are breathing too hard, you will burn more calories in the form of carbohydrate instead of breaking down unwanted fat. Here is the formula applied to a fifty-year-old:

Formula = 220 – age x .6 and .8
220 – 50 = 170
Lower Range = 170 x .6 = 102 beats per minute
Higher Range = 170 x .8 = 136 beats per minute

For me, my range to keep my body focused on burning fat is between 102 and 136 beats per minute. You can monitor your heart rate through various electronic devices, such as heart rate monitor bracelets, for as little as thirty dollars. They now have watches that also take your pulse. The old-school method of feeling your pulse for sixty seconds (or counting heartbeats on your wrist for fifteen seconds and then multiplying by four) will also work. A nice benefit on the elliptical machine I use at the gym, is that it reads your pulse through the handle grips so you can see your pulse rate as you go.

On the elliptical, I found it was easy to stay around 120, and as I got in good shape, keeping my heart rate around 130 was achievable. Maintaining this pace for an hour helped the fat burn. This same principle is easily applied to walking: walk at a pace that keeps you in the right fat-burning heart rate range.

FAT IS DIFFERENT THAN "WEIGHT"

Our goal is to lose fat, not just weight. Yes, losing fat will cause you to lose weight—at least in the short run. When you lose weight, it is almost always a combination of losing fat, muscle, and water. The more drastic and faster the weight loss, generally the more muscle and water lost. Water weight will simply be regained when you drink water or other fluids. Losing muscle is bad in both the short and long run. We want to gain muscle, which means adding weight but good weight. So, generally, slow weight loss can be a higher percentage of fat loss, which is the goal.

Historically, dieting has meant deprivation. Healthy eating is good. Food is not bad. But bad food choices add unnecessary fat over time and build an unhealthy body. You literally are what you eat.

A quick example of this is someone who loses twenty pounds in a month by eating few calories with no exercise. On the scale, they see a twenty-pound drop, but physically, this may be five pounds of fat and fifteen pounds of muscle and water. While it looks great on the scale and the person will look and be skinnier, losing muscle is bad for you and usually, if not always, ends with future weight gain. Unless you are getting body composition testing before and after, you won't know what percentage of fat or muscle you are losing, but the principle stands. Bottom line: losing muscle is not good, and that's what happens with excessively restrictive diets combined with no resistance training.

The scientific term that describes how the body breaks down muscle is called *gluconeogenesis*.

Gluconeogenesis: Glucose formation in animals from a noncarbohydrate source, as from proteins or fats.[30]

Basically, if you radically cut calories and don't exercise, your body needs to have energy to function, so it literally breaks down muscle (protein) and creates glucose (sugar), which is the body's form of carbohydrate to be used for energy. If you break down the word gluconeogenesis, it literally means "the new creation of glucose."

Gluco: for glucose or sugar
Neo: new
Genesis: creation

The problem with deprivation diets is that with insufficient protein and lack of resistance training to maintain or build muscle, you are literally breaking down the tissue you need to be healthy and burn more calories. You may temporarily win on the scale, but you set yourself up for a slower metabolism, which means carrying more fat in the days ahead. I purposely list our focus in the order of 1) build muscle, 2) burn fat, and 3) eat right because muscle is your fat-burning machine, both now and in the future. That muscle needs energy from fat to do the cardiovascular work.

BIG IDEAS

Your diet is simply what you eat.

Exercising in your target heart rate focuses on burning fat.

Your goal is not just weight loss but fat loss.

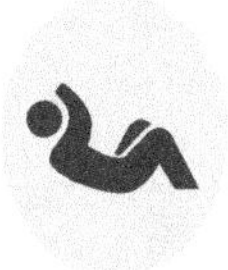

ACTION STEPS

Learn, learn, learn. The more you understand how your body functions, the simpler it will be to make right choices.

Commit to a holistic view of healthy weight that involves:

a. Cardiovascular exercise or HIIT to burn fat.

b. Resistance training to maintain/build muscle.

c. A healthy diet that provides needed nutrients and allows for weight loss or maintenance.

Learn to measure and stay within your target heart rate to purposely burn fat.

EAT RIGHT

Don't eat anything your great-grandmother wouldn't recognize as food.
—MICHAEL POLLAN[31]

I REALLY needed to work on my eating to lose weight. I eat for sport, for fun. If it's bad for you, I like it. To change, I had to be intentional with food shopping, preparation, and eating. Specifically, I had to learn about timing my meals and changing my eating patterns and choices based on my age and the way my body utilizes food differently than it did five or ten years ago. Many people work hard in the gym but don't get desired results because of food choices and the times they eat.

EAT NATURAL

Eating right begins with eating naturally, which is one of the best ways to achieve and maintain optimal bodyweight/BMI and health. Food in natural forms contains the highest nutrient levels and the least amount of negative ingredients. Generally, when food is processed, vitamins are cooked out, fiber is removed, and fat and sugar are added, along with all kinds of artificial colorings, preservatives, and other things we can't pronounce—the effects of which scientists can't fully predict.

Simply put, you must minimize or eliminate things that come in wrappers and have the word *snack* or *fast food* attached to them. I'm not someone who totally eliminates these things or gets extreme, but the less you eat of prepared, packaged, quick foods, the better.

Though more healthy prepared food options are available now than ever before, you must still diligently read the label to see what's in them. Ingredients are listed from greatest percentage by weight to least. If the number one ingredient is sugar, then corn syrup, then the top two ingredients are pure sugar. Many "health foods" are not healthy, just overpriced snacks that are one step above a candy bar.

WHAT ABOUT ENERGY DRINKS?

Like everything else, it's all about ingredients. Some of the most popular energy drinks are simply sugar-flavored water. Some of the newer ones also add a ton of caffeine. Some of the more specialized sport drinks are better, but most are overpriced drinks that give the same benefit as eating fruit and drinking a lot of water. Remember, too, anything that packs a powerful energy punch will probably have a downside when it wears off, which will encourage you to recaffeinate or eat junky snacks.

FOCUSING ON FRUITS, VEGETABLES, AND WHOLE GRAINS

Fruits and vegetables contain needed vitamins, minerals, and fiber. In an ideal world, we would never need to take vitamins or minerals because we would get optimal amounts from fruits and vegetables, which are naturally bursting with these nutrients. However, modern commercial farming often produces produce with fewer nutrients than organic or traditional methods. Fiber also packs many health benefits, in addition to helping us feel fuller longer, meaning we're less likely to overeat or eat junk food.

VARIETY AND AMOUNTS

Again, simple math: the greater the variety and volume of fruits and vegetables, the richer and more diverse supply of nutrients received. Try to eat as much organic and/or fresh produce as possible. Organic produce has more nutrients due to healthier soil management techniques, such as using nutrient-rich fertilizers instead of chemical fertilizers, which don't resupply the soil with needed nutrients.

Your next best option, if you can't get or afford organics, is buying local produce that can be picked further along in the ripening process when greater nutrients abound. Short transit time means fewer preservatives are used and more nutrients are maintained.

CONSISTENTLY ADD FRUITS AND VEGETABLES

In my weight maintenance stage, I packed my bag of "rabbit food" when I had to work late. This was basically a one-gallon plastic bag of three carrots, three celery stalks, and a half of a cucumber chopped up and eaten from seven to ten o'clock to satisfy hunger without resorting to eating junk food. The more you can make this standard a habit, the better.

BAKE, BBQ, OR BOIL INSTEAD OF FRY

When you fry meat, you are coating it and cooking it in fat, which greatly increases the food's fat and calorie count. Yes, I love fried foods, and yes, I eat them, but I try to limit them. When you bake, BBQ, or boil, you are not adding unneeded fat but instead adding flavor through seasoning and the cooking process. When you add natural spices and take the time to cook it slowly, the food will be healthier. You can also prepare a salad while the meat is cooking.

Boiled eggs can also be a good protein choice because of the high-protein, low-calorie ratio in egg whites. Generally, I will eat the egg white and throw out the yolk because that's where the fat and cholesterol are. Eating egg whites, either as part of your meal or as a snack between meals, adds low-calorie protein to your diet, and they're easy to make and bring with you.

CHOOSING HEALTHY MEATS AND FISH

Recent healthy diet trends focus on eating clean. These regiments recommend natural and organic meats and fish. Wild fish will be cleaner and healthier than farm raised. Meat raised without hormones and antibiotics will best conventionally raised meat. Limiting and staying away from cold cuts, sausage, and bacon is also prudent. As far as trendy diets go, Paleo is probably the healthiest and most practical for people to follow as it also includes fruits, vegetables, nuts, seeds, and healthy oils.

WHAT ABOUT KETO DIETS?

High-fat, moderate-protein, no-carb diets have been around for a while. Before the keto diet, a similar version was the Atkins diet, and there have been others. A standard keto diet would get its calories from the following:

Fat: 60-75 percent
Protein: 20-25 percent
Carbs: 5-10 percent

I've never been a fan of these diets for several reasons. The biggest reason is that, for most people, the effects don't last. These approaches work because they suppress the production of insulin, which is an effective way to lose weight, but like most quick solution diets, once you start eating normally again, the weight and then some comes back. Yes, they can be effective, but most people will end up in worse shape than when they started. You are choosing an unnatural way of eating that is not sustainable over time.

Next, they also produce a pretty high toxicity level in your body, which is why so much water is recommended to avoid damaging your kidneys. Weight loss on these plans can be dramatic and quick but unhealthy in both the short and long term. Increased exercise routines and knowledge has made these types of diets more effective, both short and long term.

MY MODIFIED KETO/CARB CYCLING/INTERMITTENT FASTING EXPERIENCE

While I spent over a year losing twenty-three pounds using the traditional approach of healthier eating and increased exercise, I did implement a modified keto diet, combined with carb cycling and intermittent fasting, for the last four weeks. This change helped me drop the last seventeen pounds. I was comfortable using this more radical method for a short amount of time because I'd spent over a year building my health.

I went on an all-protein and fat diet on Monday, Wednesday, and Friday, meaning no carbs on these days and only eating between noon and eight o'clock in the evening. Then I added fruits and vegetables on the other four weekdays to replenish vitamins, minerals, and other nutrients. After the final four-week sprint, I immediately went back to a more balanced diet to ensure my body didn't go into too much stress and shock and then bounce back with weight gain.

Personally, this time-limited effort had great results without overly stressing my body or slowing down my metabolism. The downside was that my cholesterol jumped up to 267 at the end of the four weeks, so I had to focus on decreasing that number after my modified keto sprint.

NO SILVER BULLETS, MAGIC FOODS, OR EASY FIXES

One thing I keep in mind is that weight gain and weight loss are simple processes that happen over time. Quick solutions rarely last and usually create a slower metabolism and increased future weight gain.

No special food can melt away fat either. Years ago, the grapefruit diet promised weight loss if people lived on grapefruits. Of course, devotees dropped pounds because they had drastically reduced caloric intake by only eating grapefruit; it's math, not a miracle. This diet works as long as you never eat anything but grapefruit again. I won't address the million other diets that have come and gone since the grapefruit diet, but beware of any diet that promises fast results or easy fixes.

BENEFITS OF INCREASED FIBER BY FOCUSING ON VEGETABLES AND WHOLE GRAIN

Following is information and data from the Mayo Clinic article "Dietary Fiber: Essential for a Healthy Diet":[32]

Healthy Benefits of Increased Fiber Include:
1. Maintaining healthy bodyweight
2. Longer life expectancy through lowering risk of
   - Heart disease
   - Diabetes
   - Some types of cancer
3. Normalized bowel movements relieving constipation

4. Lower cholesterol
5. More stabilized blood sugar levels

Different Types of Dietary Fiber

Fiber is commonly classified as soluble, which dissolves in water, or insoluble, which doesn't dissolve.

Soluble Fiber: This type of fiber dissolves in water to form a gel-like material. It can help lower blood cholesterol and glucose levels. Soluble fiber is found in oats, peas, beans, apples, citrus fruits, carrots, barley, and psyllium.

Insoluble Fiber: This type of fiber promotes the movement of material through your digestive system and increases stool bulk, so it can be of benefit to those who struggle with constipation or irregular stools. Whole-wheat flour, wheat bran, nuts, beans, and vegetables, such as cauliflower, green beans, and potatoes, are good sources of insoluble fiber.

Eat These to Increase Fiber Intake:

1. Whole grain foods: Try oatmeal, breads, pasta, etc. Avoid refined or processed versions.
2. Whole fruits and vegetables: Eat raw, homemade juices that keep fiber. Avoid canned or processed versions.
3. Beans, peas, and legumes
4. Nuts and seeds (in limited amounts)

DON'T FORGET THE BIG PICTURE

Remember, our goal is not just to lose weight but to lose fat and be healthy. Eating a natural, high-fiber diet has many short- and long-term effects. My goal of hitting 190 pounds was not to be cute on my fiftieth birthday but to set the standard for how I want to feel at sixty, seventy, eighty, and ninety. If I weigh 190 on my fiftieth birthday but 230 on my fifty-second, that is failure, not success. I don't want to be that eighty-year-old guy sitting in a rocking chair trying to keep track of whether I took all my meds for the day. I tend to be a playful person, so every once in a while, I will tell people who are younger than me that when I am jogging by the nursing home they will be in, I will stop and visit. They tell me that won't happen, and I smile and say, "See you then!"

DRINK MORE WATER

Drinking water is like washing out your insides. The water will cleanse the system, fill you up, decrease your caloric load, and improve the function of all your tissues. –KEVIN R. STONE [33]

After air, the most important thing a person needs to survive is water. You can only live a few minutes without air and a few days without water, but you can live for weeks without food.

HOW MUCH WATER SHOULD I DRINK?

The standard recommendation and starting point is that everyone should drink eight glasses of eight ounces of water each day (sixty-four ounces total). This is a basic recommendation for health. The amount increases if someone is larger than normal or exercising, which causes increased sweating and, therefore, increases the need for water. We should look at the traditional sixty-four-ounce recommendation as a base minimum for the average person. Someone who is 250 pounds, working out an hour a day, or in a hotter climate will need more water to maintain healthy hydration.

HOW DO I KNOW IF I AM GETTING ENOUGH WATER?

The easiest way to know if you are getting enough water is by observing your urine. Sounds exciting, doesn't it? It's simple. Do you urinate frequently? Urinating six to eight times a day is normal, but frequency is affected by the amount of fluids you drink, and caffeine will also make you urinate more frequently. What does your urine look and smell like? No, you don't have to get too close. If it is clear, fairly odorless, and large in volume, you are better hydrated than if it is dark, has a stronger smell, and is low volume.

A better goal, especially if you are large, sweating during workouts, and trying to lose weight, is to drink between one half to one ounce of water per pound of bodyweight. So, a two-hundred-pound person should aim for one hundred to two hundred ounces of water per day.

What does that look like? Personally, I put a twelve-ounce glass of water on my dresser. I would drink a little before I went to bed, have a sip if I woke up at all in the night, and drink anything left in the morning. This started me off with twelve ounces of water each day. During my workout, I drank a forty-ounce bottle. I would then fill that bottle one or two more times per day for a total of ninety-two to 132 ounces of water per day. Most water bottles are sixteen ounces. I keep a case of water in the trunk of my car. If you drink six bottles of sixteen ounces per day, that is ninety-six ounces. These totals will help keep you healthy and clean along your weight loss and maintenance journey.

DOES DRINKING WATER MAKE YOU LOSE FAT?

The short answer is no, drinking water doesn't *make* you lose fat in the sense that it does not directly cause weight loss. Water has zero calories, meaning it does not add calories or energy to your body. So if you drink more water, it will not cause weight loss in the same way walking or jogging an extra mile can. That being said, water keeps your body clean and functioning at an optimal level. Having sufficient water can makes a positive difference in how you feel and how your body functions, causing your other weight-loss efforts to have a greater effect.

CAN DRINKING WATER HELP YOU LOSE FAT?

One hundred percent yes. When part of an overall health plan, drinking water can *help* you lose fat. How does that work?

ZERO CALORIES IS LESS THAN ANY AMOUNT OF CALORIES

Since water has zero calories, every time you drink it instead of juice, soda, alcohol, or any drink with calories, you have removed the intake of unnecessary calories. Brilliant, right? I am not saying never to drink juice, soda, or alcohol, but let's go back to the math. A case of soda or beer has enough calories to add one pound of fat if you don't burn the extra calories off. *Beer belly* is a term for a reason; guys who drink beer and don't burn it off get a belly. It's not complex.

NO INSULIN IS RELEASED FROM WATER

Remember that when our blood sugar hits a certain level, the body releases insulin, which stores some of the sugar and fat. So, no sugar added means less insulin released and that means less fat storage. This is a physiological process that mechanically responds according to our body's design. Simply put, our body will burn more of the calories we eat when we drink water with meals and store more as fat when we drink sugary drinks with our meals. It's the same food intake, but our body deals with it better when we drink water. So, it's a double benefit when we drink water with meals; it removes unnecessary calories and decreases insulin production and the fat-storing process.

PROPER HYDRATION HELPS YOUR METABOLISM WORK BETTER

Dehydration by as little as 1 percent can cause metabolism to function less efficiently. Essentially, just as an engine needs oil to function at peak efficiency, your body needs sufficient water to work at peak efficiency.[34]

GIVE YOUR INSIDES A BATH

Most people enjoy a daily shower to keep their body clean. Every day, we sweat, secrete oils, and inadvertently pick up germs and dirt. A hot shower strips all this away and makes us feel better. I look at the water I drink in a similar way: every glass of water I drink washes my insides. The water we drink first helps us function at our peak. And what we excrete through sweat, urine, and water vapor (as we breathe) is ridding the body of used-up nutrients or part of your food or body that has been broken down and is essentially toxic if not properly excreted.

DRINKING WATER BEFORE A MEAL CAN MAKE YOU EAT LESS

One study showed that people who drank a glass of water before a meal ate seventy-five calories less at each meal. If someone simply drank water before dinner every day for a year, twenty-seven thousand calories (eight pounds) would be avoided. Do that for three years and a person could avoid gaining, and even possibly lose, about twenty-five pounds of fat. That is a significant effect for such a small change.

HEADACHES AND FATIGUE

Part of my job is to solve people's problems. When anyone tells me they are either tired or have a headache, my go-to response is, "Have you tried drinking a big glass of water?" The answer is almost always no. Usually, when I see them later, they will smile and say thank you because that water made them feel better.

When your body doesn't have enough water, it lets you know in all kinds of ways, including headache and fatigue. Your body simply functions better with proper hydration. If headache or fatigue are caused by other things, then water will not make them go away, but you would be surprised at how often a glass or bottle of water can make a person feel better. So, if you want to feel your best every day, then properly hydrate.

BIG IDEAS

Eat foods that are closest to their natural state
(their least cooked/processed form) and drink at least
sixty-four ounces of pure water daily.

High-fiber foods have great health benefits.

Short-term keto diets can be effective but should not replace
a long-term health plan.

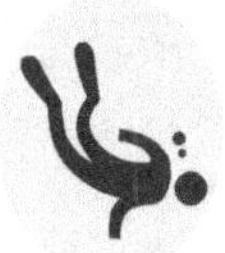

ACTION STEPS

Substitute healthy, natural foods for processed, packaged foods.

Integrate high-fiber foods into your daily food schedule.

Plan to drink a minimum of sixty-four ounces of water daily with a goal of one half to one ounce of water per pound of bodyweight.

SCHEDULE WORKOUTS

Excuses are for people that don't want it bad enough.[35]

For years, I was lazy or too busy, so I skipped going to the gym. Something always pulls on our time unless we are deliberate. Scheduling workouts and keeping them as a priority increased my weight-loss progress.

TREAT YOUR WORKOUTS LIKE AN IMPORTANT MEETING

Imagine you're up for a promotion after you present at a meeting or that you have a lunch appointment to cut the next big deal. Would you skip either because you were too busy or a little tired? No way! Would you skip a date with the one you had been looking for and think you finally found? Not a chance!

So, you want me to treat my next workout like it is that important?

Yes! If you want success in your fat-loss and energy-increase plan, you must see your workouts as essential. Imagine you had a month to submit a proposal that would literally change your life. I guarantee you that, for that month, you would be focused on that proposal every extra moment. You would get up early and stay up late—without question. That's what people do when things are important to them. So, what does this look like in terms of our workouts?

Make Workouts Non-negotiable in Your Mind

Don't give yourself any wiggle room. If you plan a workout, don't change it—unless you have a legit, one-time emergency. Discipline yourself not to make excuses or live sloppily. You can always find some reason that is "important." Don't open the door to that type of thinking. You should have a priority list of things to do each day that are non-negotiable, things that will have the greatest return or make your life better. Working out needs to be on that list. Then you are ready for the next step.

Put Workouts in Your Phone, aka "Assign Time to Your Priorities"

Assigning chunks of time to your established priorities is one of the best disciplines to improve your life. Put your workout in your phone calendar like any other important, nonnegotiable appointment. You may choose before work, after work, or even at lunchtime, but once the workout slot is in your phone, stick to it.

When people ask me to have a phone conference or meet during the timeslot my workout is scheduled in my phone, I simply tell them I have another appointment at that time and give them several other times that are open. I don't hurt my professional or private life, and I follow through on my commitment to health. This can be emotionally challenging at first, but once you build the habit and see the benefit, it becomes a no-brainer.

DILIGENCE AND DISCIPLINE

Building muscle, burning fat, and eating right never happen by accident. By scheduling workouts, you are building your "diligence and discipline muscles." When you schedule and keep workouts, you train both your body and mind to achieve your health goals. Progress comes when you repetitively apply a few basic principles over time.

FREEDOM BY PRACTICING DISCIPLINE

Discipline equals freedom. –JOCKO WILLINK[36]

One of the books I read while writing this book was called *Extreme Ownership*. It taught that the more you create order and discipline in your life, the greater control and freedom you will have with the rest of your life.

By disciplining yourself to plan your workout, put it in your phone, and show up at the gym, track, or Zumba® class, you will gain the freedom to be healthy, feel better, and live better. Developing the discipline to say no to people who want to eat away at your time allows you to be the person you were created to be, instead of some overweight, tired, and broken-down person with no energy or passion for life.

GREATER EMOTIONAL STABILITY AND LESS ANXIETY

Order brings stability. Anxiety is caused when you feel either overwhelmed or out of control. If I *might* work out later today, every phone call, interruption, or person who wants "just a minute" brings stress as

I watch my workout time get slowly eaten away. If I already worked out in the morning or on my lunch break or had it locked into my schedule for after work, I won't feel the anxiety of choosing what to do. When it's time to go to the gym, it's time to go to the gym. This surety brings a sense of control because I am in control. I have a calendar on my phone that I created, and it orders my life to achieve my goals.

SIMPLE BUT POWERFUL

It's so funny that the more degrees I get and the smarter and more experienced I become, the more I realize that the most powerful things in life are often the simplest. For example, commitment is merely a yes or no, but it is powerful. Consider NBA basketball players who shoot one hundred foul shots every day to make that skill second nature, so they'll know what to do automatically when they are called upon in a game. Likewise, once you know what to do for your health and you do it repetitively over time, you will get the benefit or reward you want. Your progress will increase when you make your workouts nonnegotiable.

BIG IDEAS

Treat your workouts like important meetings you can't skip.

If something is important, you will assign time to it.

Discipline will get you more freedom.

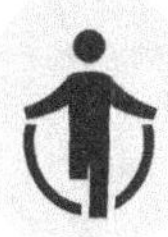

ACTION STEPS

Make your workouts non-negotiable.

Put your workouts in your phone.

Show up and work out. Treat it like an important business or personal appointment you must keep.

JUST LOSE ONE POUND

Success is the sum of small efforts, repeated day in and day out.
—ROBERT COLLIER [37]

I used small wins to stay motivated. Setting goals and achieving them encouraged me to repeat my efforts. Losing thirty-five pounds seemed like a forever process because I was committed to doing it in a healthy and sustainable way. To stay motivated along the way, I deliberately weighed myself once a week on Friday mornings, with the goal to see one pound less on the scale. This gave me a full week to work to lose that pound. It also gave me Monday to Friday to burn off anything extra I ate over the weekend.

KEEP IT SIMPLE

Losing weight is super simple: burn more calories than you eat over time and you will lose weight. Period. Easy to understand but often hard to do; otherwise, no one would have excess fat. When people ask me the secret to losing weight, I smile and tell them to buy a pair of sneakers and jog three to five days a week. Come back to me when the sneakers are worn out, and you will have lost weight. Simple, right? Get rid of the candy bars, chips, and soda, and it will happen even faster. But when you have people like me who hate running and love snacking, the simple becomes more complex.

Yes, other factors like metabolic rate, conditioning, and hormone levels affect how the body modulates fat level, but at the end of the day, fat is stored energy that we measure in calories.

WHICH DIET IS BEST?

You will not find a super diet in this book but a discussion on habits. I recommend a lifestyle based on healthy nutrition principles. The true definition of the word *diet* is simple: what you eat. When we hear the word *diet*, we often think of a strict regimen or some type of deprivation leading to weight loss. These approaches can be effective in losing weight short term, but they often backfire when it comes to long-term health and weight management. Our focus will be on making positive, lasting changes that become part of our everyday life.

ANYONE CAN LOSE A POUND OF FAT

*A year from now you will wish you had started today. —*KAREN LAMB[38]

Remember, just start. You can do this. Lose one pound—that's burning thirty-five hundred unused calories stored within the body. Fat is part of everyone's body. In fact, every person has a good amount of fat, and a certain amount is even needed.

According to the American Counsel of Exercise (ACE), the average six-foot man has an acceptable fat percentage between 18-24 percent.[39] This means the average two-hundred-pound man will have between thirty-six and forty-eight pounds of fat. Add thirty pounds of fat gained over time, and you are looking at sixty-six to seventy-eight pounds of fat. So, the average guy walking around with the dad bod may be carrying seventy-five pounds of fat. Fat is not evil or bad. It makes babies cute and adds beauty to women, but excess fat is detrimental to overall health and daily energy levels.

Another way to measure fat is the body mass index (BMI), which is a height to weight ratio. Let me share my results—though it's not exact science. When I started at 228 pounds (at six feet), my BMI was 30.9, with obesity starting at 30. After weight loss, when I was at 188 pounds, my BMI was 25.4, which is considered slightly overweight (24.9 or lower is considered normal).[40] I took my journey one pound at a time and so can you.

THE PROBLEM OF EXCESS FAT

How easy is it to gain one pound of fat? Remember, it's thirty-five hundred extra calories that were eaten but not burned off. What does this look like in the real world?

If you eat an extra five hundred calories per day that is not burned off, you will add one pound of fat in a week. Another way to look at it is that if you eat an extra one hundred calories per day for five weeks, you will gain one pound of fat. Simply eating an extra one hundred calories per day will cause you to gain ten pounds of fat in a year. It is easy to see how the weight can creep on.

Same thing works in reverse. If you remove something unnecessary, like an afternoon soda, it adds up over time. One can of soda is one hundred fifty calories. One case of soda is twenty-four cans: 24 x 150 = 3,600 calories or one pound of fat. If you replaced a daily can of soda with a bottle of water and changed nothing else, you could drop over one pound of fat per month (twelve pounds in a year).

IT'S MATH

Every day, you either gain or lose fat based on your activity and diet. Think of it like a bank account. If every dollar represents a calorie, one pound of fat would be thirty-five hundred dollars in the bank. Just like you would either deposit or withdraw money over time, we add or subtract fat on our bodies over time.

WALKING ONE MILE BURNS ABOUT ONE HUNDRED CALORIES FOR A ONE HUNDRED EIGHTY-POUND PERSON

Walking one mile will burn about one hundred calories if you weigh one hundred eighty pounds. You'll burn more if you weigh more and less if you way less, but let's use the one hundred-calorie amount for our discussion. So, if you skipped that can of soda, instead grabbed a water bottle, and walked two miles, your efforts would produce a net loss of three hundred fifty calories and add up to one pound of fat in ten days or three pounds of fat in one month. That would be thirty-six pounds in a year. This is about small decisions and actions adding up over time. If you were in the gym building muscle at the same time, you would burn more calories as you walk. Bottom line: you can do this.

DAMAGE CAUSED BY CARRYING EXCESSIVE FAT

Added Stress on Your Heart

Every pound of fat requires additional blood circulation, meaning the body must build new and additional blood vessels called *capillaries*. Scientists say that every pound of fat has approximately one mile of capillaries, and your heart must pump blood through these extra blood vessels.[41] Because I lost forty pounds of fat, I now have about forty fewer miles of capillaries for my heart to push blood through. My heart is saying thank you.

The reason you take an elevator instead of walking up ten to twenty flights of stairs is because those stairs are stressful. With forty extra miles of blood vessels to work with, my heart must have felt like it was walking up stairs even when I was sitting at my desk. Every pound of fat you lose will make your heart smile.

Clogged Arteries

It is common knowledge that excess triglycerides and cholesterol in our blood vessels lead to clogged arteries over time. This leads to increased rates of high blood pressure, heart attacks, and strokes. In fact, we know it and hear it so many times that we become numb to it. While we are numb and overweight, guess what? Your blood vessels are slowly clogging up.

Stress on Your Joints

Your joints absorb the stress of movement. Between bones is shock-absorber tissue called cartilage. Every time you take a step, whether walking or jogging, your hips, knees, and feet must absorb the shock of each and every step. Shock increases with increased weight. I have heard about foot pain in people who are fifty or one hundred pounds overweight. In addition to cartilage, ligaments attach bone to bone. So, imagine your feet being stressed with every step and pulling on the ligaments between bones. These can become sprained, stretched, or even torn because of the excessive stress placed on them from walking. Stress from jogging or higher impact movements could be worse.

It's easy to see how a cycle of weight gain and poor health is perpetuated. If your feet or joints hurt, you will exercise less and either maintain or gain weight. If you gain weight, your feet or joints will hurt more, so you will want to do even less. These downward cycles are broken when we start to lose weight and take pressure off our feet and joints so we can exercise more, lose more weight, and feel better. Every pound lost means less stress on your body.

Increased Lower Back Pain

Excessive abdominal fat is one of the most common causes of lower back pain. Our spine has a natural curve. Excessive abdominal fat causes the natural spinal curve to become exaggerated, causing nerves to be pinched and muscles to be stressed and pulled. This results in lower back pain and muscle spasms.

Back pain can also make exercise more difficult if back muscles are tight, weak, or stretched out. As you will see throughout this book, one problem often creates another. Excessive body fat causes back pain resulting in decreased exercise leading to more weight gain. More weight gain then causes more back pain, and this can be an ongoing cycle. In the same way, as we lose weight, strengthen muscles, and increase flexibility, a healthier cycle develops.

FAT LOSS HAS GREAT BENEFITS

The statistics are undeniable. With increased body fat percentages, rates of high blood pressure, heart disease, diabetes, strokes, arthritis, and even cancer will increase. If excess fat increases the risk and occurrence of all these, then fat loss decreases their risk and occurrence. No one would purposely sign up for these ailments, but we literally invite them into our lives when we carry excess fat. One way to stay motivated is to think that every pound of weight lost decreases the risk of all these things.

LET'S GET RID OF ONE POUND OF FAT

One pound of fat is thirty-five hundred calories. If you burn five hundred extra calories per day for one week, it will add up to one pound in a week. Here are a couple more examples:

Day 1: Walk two miles to burn 200 calories; drink two glasses of water instead of two sodas to save 300 calories = 500 calorie deficit

Day 2: Go to gym and do 20 minutes of elliptical (200 calories), 30 minutes of resistance training (150 calories); to eliminate 340 calories, eat an apple (80 calories) and drink water instead of having a small bag of potato chips (270 calories) and a soda (150 calories) = 690 calorie deficit

Day 3: Walk one mile (burn 100 calories); to save 460 calories, replace a Big Mac meal (1,100 calories)[42] with a Panera turkey sandwich on whole grain bread (560 calories)[43] with an apple (80 calories) = 560 calorie deficit

In three days, these small changes would result in a negative calorie balance of 1,750 calories. Repeat the same pattern to lose 3,500 calories in six days. That's one pound of fat gone. You can do this, but it takes intentional, consistent effort.

Remember, I am not a big calorie counter. I share these numbers to demonstrate the power of right choices over time. One of my best changes was eliminating unnecessary snacks or purposely snacking on raw fruits or vegetables.

Losing fat will make you feel better. You'll have less pain while increasing your daily energy levels. Just stay focused on losing that next pound.

BIG IDEAS

Anyone can lose a pound of fat.

It's math. If you burn more calories than you eat each day, then over time you will lose weight.

Increased fat causes health problems; decreased fat reduces them.

ACTIONS

Consider how you can decrease unnecessary calories (i.e., drink water instead of sugary soda or juice).

Reduce or eliminate unhealthy fast foods. Either make or buy better options.

In addition to scheduled workouts, purposely climb stairs and walk throughout the day.

CLEAN YOUR BODY

You are what you eat.

I really need to stay focused on my food choices. Unless I purposefully discipline myself, I will eat just about anything and lots of it. I'm definitely more on the junk food side of the healthy-minded/junk-food-loving continuum. When on a roll, I can live on fast food and junk food and not feel bad about it. But to reach my goal, I seriously needed to increase my discipline and clean out my body. I did it and saw great results.

YOU ARE WHAT YOU EAT

"You are what you eat" is one of those sayings everyone knows but ignores because "everyone knows." Good or bad, the food we eat literally becomes our cells and tissues. Eating highly processed foods combined with excessive stress makes the body toxic or "dirty," which results in our body working insufficiently. Exercising, drinking lots of water, and decreasing stress cleans our internal body. Eating clean means eating simple, natural foods that the body can easily digest and utilize to build health.

DON'T GET SCARED BY EXTREME PEOPLE

Over the years, I've met extreme people who are always cleansing by following some strange program; that's not what I am talking about. I am 100 percent in line with eating, drinking, and exercising in ways that keep our body clean without resorting to strange supplements or super strict food regiments. It doesn't take extended fasts or purging methods to live and eat clean.

If someone wants to go vegan, or at least increase vegetables while reducing meat or processed foods, this is wise and sustainable. If someone leans toward the paleo diet (unprocessed foods, clean meats, etc.), that's a good move. But if you tell me I have to drink twelve glasses of celery juice and go to the bathroom fourteen times a day and sit in a sauna until I'm about to faint, I'm walking away.

LET'S CLEAN UP THAT DIET

Much has been said recently about eating clean. The idea behind this is that the cleaner the fuel, the better and more efficiently your body will work. As your body functions better, you will feel better. In the same way your car works better with clean motor oil, transmission oil, and air and auto filters, the better your body will run the cleaner your blood and organs (liver, kidneys, intestines).

WHAT ARE CLEAN FOODS?

Clean foods are simply foods in their natural state, like pure water, fruits, vegetables, lean meat, and fish. Natural seasonings are used to give flavor instead of relying on deep-frying. For several months of my weight-loss journey, I drank only water, black coffee, and fresh vegetable juice. Because I was not eating sugars, fried foods, or thick gravies and sauces, my enjoyment of fruits and vegetables was enhanced. I started eating whole carrots, which tasted better than candy to me.

TIPS FOR EATING CLEAN

Eat Whole Foods in the Simplest Forms

Raw fruits and vegetables can be eaten as part of your meals or snacks or you can make juice and drink them. One guideline is to eat fruits and drink vegetables. Why? Fruit is easy to eat, especially as snacks, to provide a pick-me-up and sustained energy throughout the day. Vegetables are harder to eat in volume and variety, but you can quickly drink carrot, spinach, and ginger in a drink. I have a Vitamix® at home and a Nutri Ninja® at my office. I try to have a vegetable-based drink at least once a day. My most common combo is one carrot, one apple, spinach or kale, and ginger. I also tend to juice grapefruits because this fruit is easier to drink than eat whole.

Limit Highly Processed and Packaged Food

While studying nutrition at Columbia University, I often heard, "Don't eat it if it comes in a wrapper." That was over twenty years ago. Now, some "healthy" foods come in a wrapper, but the principle remains. Generally, the more people mess with food, the more unhealthy it becomes—unless they are going out of their way to package a healthy food.

In addition, many "health" foods are not necessarily healthy. Read labels. Ingredients are listed from highest to lowest contribution. If sugar is the number one ingredient, it's more plentiful than any other ingredient, contributing a significant amount of empty calories. Many energy bars are high-priced candy bars filled with sugar or high fructose corn syrup. If the ingredients are good, eat it. If the ingredients are the same as a candy bar, then you may as well eat the candy bar.

UNCLEAN FOODS

Unclean foods are highly processed foods that are fried or contain excessive salt, sugar, chemical preservatives, or white flour. Unclean foods have been highly altered from their natural state and often contain additives a person would never eat if packaged with more transparency.

When a company produces a product, their main goal is to sell as many units as possible to make money. As a capitalist, I agree with the idea of profit, but I also know most people are tempted to buy foods that taste good, regardless of the item's nutrition. So, it's easy to eat unhealthy foods because salt, sugar, fat, and other chemical additives make these foods taste better and last longer. Unless a company has a vision to produce healthy foods, their goal is to produce good-tasting products that sell.

Our body must process all these added unhealthy ingredients, causing stress on our organs, clogging our arteries, and raising our blood pressure. Also, as our blood sugar spikes, our pancreas is overworked. Our kidneys and heart work harder as our hydration levels are affected by excessive salt, and our poor liver has to filter out the chemicals and preservatives. Our stomachs have to digest unnatural products man was not designed to eat.

I used to remind my kids to close snack and cereal bags tightly, but I stopped when I realized that these foods don't go stale if you leave them open. Who knows what these preservatives are doing to food quality and our bodies?

PREPARE YOUR OWN FOODS

If you make your own food, then you know exactly what's in it. Yes, this takes time, but it ensures you are eating what you want. Our culture makes it easy to live on fast and prepared foods. This is one of the areas where behavior is more important than knowledge. We know that ninety-nine cent cheeseburgers are not optimal nutrition, but if you are like me, you opt for easy over healthy too often.

Consider breakfast. If I make oatmeal for breakfast each day and drink black coffee, I tend to maintain or lose weight. If I don't make oatmeal, I pick up some type of breakfast sandwich and drink coffee with milk and sugar—and I gain weight. This creates a cycle of being tired, picking up fast food, and gaining weight, which leads to being tired and repeating the same behavior the next day. When I take the time to make my food, I eat better and feel better.

PACKING LUNCH, SNACKS, JUICES FOR WORK

When I pack my lunch on workdays, I not only eat better, but I also set the tone for my day. Intentionally packing healthy options helps me stay focused and not slide into bad habits while away from home.

Truth is, I will cheat on eating healthy in the name of getting things done at work. If I don't have healthy snacks and juices throughout the day, I also will visit my coworker who has a bowl of chocolate on her desk. If I don't prepare properly, I will end up eating a handful (or two) of chocolate snacks or grabbing a fast-food lunch so I can power through.

EATING CLEAN BRINGS MENTAL CLARITY AND FOCUS

Eating clean helps us think clearly; it allows greater focus because it keeps our blood sugar levels more stable. The brain uses carbohydrates to get energy to function. When our blood sugar is low, our brains don't function as well. Instinctively we know this, and this is why we unconsciously reach for junk food. We know it works. That chocolate bar or cookie will give my brain the sugar it needs to function.

In addition to aiding thinking and the processing of information, normalized blood sugar from consuming healthy foods helps stabilize emotions and equips us to respond to people better. Currently, I have three teenagers and a preteen in my house. At times they tell each other to get something to eat because one of them is *hangry*. This means they are hungry and angry at the same time. They know that the cure to agitation is often food.

Instead of using junk food to boost our blood sugar levels, eat clean, which will keep your levels in a healthy range all throughout the day. Eating clean keeps our blood clean of unnatural additives, which results in increased energy and feelings of well-being.

HEALTHY TRENDING

We often trend either in a good or bad direction in our habits and life. When it comes to eating, we either trend toward healthy choices or unhealthy. Like I said, if I start with oatmeal and black coffee and continue my day with vegetable juicing, water, and fruit, everything trends toward healthy. I also work out more when I'm eating well. The opposite trend is eating junk food and then skipping my workout. Clearly, we want to intentionally foster positive cycles that not only produce physical health but also support mental clarity and emotional health.

TWO DRINKS THAT HELPED CLEAN ME UP

Along the way, I add two different drinks to my day for a couple of months:

1. Water with lime: I squeezed a full lime into sixteen ounces of water. Lime adds vitamin C and increases blood alkalinity.

2. Ginger, turmeric, lemon juice, and honey: In a Vitamix®, blend eight ounces of water, about one inch of ginger, one piece of turmeric, juice from a whole lemon, and a little honey for thirty seconds. Pour into a twenty-five-ounce bottle and add water until full. This provides all the cleansing and anti-inflammatory benefits of ginger and turmeric with vitamin C from lemon. Honey is for taste.

These tasty creations helped me drink five cups (forty ounces) of water. Plus, I got the benefits of a whole lime and whole lemon's vitamin C and the benefits of ginger and turmeric. These beverages replaced sugary soda for me when I worked later at night. I got the double benefit of eliminating acidic, toxic ingredients in other drinks and adding in these alkaline, healthy drinks. It's a simple win-win that increased my daily energy as my body got cleaner.

BIG IDEAS

Eat raw fruits and vegetables (whole or juiced)
frequently throughout the day.

Limit highly processed foods to eat foods as close
to their natural state as possible.

Clean foods include water, raw fruits and vegetables,
whole grains, and lean meat/fish cooked without excessive oil or salt.

ACTION STEPS

Prepare your own foods and drinks. Experiment with cooking new healthy foods.

Choose healthy options when at a store or restaurant.

Stick with healthy eating long enough to see your taste buds become more sensitive, and you will enjoy simple foods more.

BUILD MOMENTUM

*An object at rest stays at rest and an object in motion
stays in motion with the same speed and in the same direction
unless acted upon by an unbalanced force.*
—Newton's first law of motion[44]

I was stuck for many years. If I had any momentum, it was negative and going in the wrong direction. To change this, I purposely planned things that would create positive momentum. I knew it would take a lot of effort in the beginning, but I trusted it would get easier once my metabolism kicked in and my body was set to build muscle and burn fat. The hardest work took place in the beginning as the benefits grew over time.

Newton's first law, the law of inertia, says if something is not moving, a strong force is required to make it move. Once something is moving, it tends to stay moving and will keep moving with little added force. So, if you are fat (sorry, trying to help) and have been sitting still, it will take more force to get you and your metabolism going. You are that force. But once you get moving and start burning fat, it will become easier over time.

One of the keys to losing and keeping weight off is to build and maintain momentum. Life has seasons; things shift. I have embraced the term *trends* to describe shifts in life's momentum. Different seasons trend in different directions. An example of such a shift is spending versus saving: the momentum to either build wealth or incur debt. Outside of some strange event, you don't wake up one day suddenly bankrupt or rich. Chances are, you will trend in one direction, usually for years, before you reach one extreme or the other.

Likewise, life satisfaction or dissatisfaction doesn't usually happen in an instant. Your level of fulfillment is a result of an ongoing series of events that pushes you toward either destination. Similarly, you don't gain or lose twenty to forty pounds in a day. It happens over months and years as you trend in one direction or another.

SHIFT FROM DRUDGERY TO FUN

Whenever I have taken time off from the gym and put on a few pounds, it is often drudgery to start again. This can be discouraging. What used to be easy is now hard. Yesterday's workout is now painful during and after. It takes time to work through this reality. With each exercise session, things become easier and more enjoyable. Finally, we want to exercise again. A momentum change happens when we go from dreading the gym to feeling like we've missed out if we skip a workout. Our diets trend or build momentum as we go from eating erratically, snacking on junk food, and eating insufficient fruits and vegetables to eating three regular meals, planning healthy snacks in between, and making water our main drink.

These trends can build both physical and psychological momentum that makes it easier to continue losing weight and keep it off. Like a car rolling downhill, we can build momentum creating greater results from our actions and choices. This momentum helps us shift from weight loss as drudgery to an enjoyable effort we look forward to.

In addition to increased muscle and decreased fat, our body can undergo biochemical changes, including increased fat-burning enzymes, increased sensitivity to insulin, and the release of endorphins in our brains.

BUILD PSYCHOLOGICAL MOMENTUM

Getting and staying in the right mind space is probably the most important aspect of losing and keeping weight off. It's not so much about what you know but about how you consistently act upon that knowledge that counts.

A positive mental attitude sets the right tone for every decision and every action. Losing weight requires many choices that may go against natural inclination or current mood. Your mental positivity must be stronger than negative feelings and pressures that will push you to eat too much or the wrong foods at the wrong times.

When your passion and desire is to eat junk food or skip your exercise session, your internal motivation and drive for continued progress must outweigh those desires. Your psychological momentum must be a greater force than the resistance or temptations you face.

Momentum also makes it easier to steer. If you have ever tried to turn the wheel of your car when the car is still, it is difficult. But when you are moving, it is easier to turn the wheel and steer the car. The faster the car movement, the greater the momentum and the easier to steer. The greater your emotional and psychological momentum, the easier for you to steer your actions toward healthy food choices and exercise levels. Every day, we must choose to build and maintain a positive attitude because we have a goal and vision of a better reality.

BUILD PHYSIOLOGICAL MOMENTUM

This idea may be new to you, but we have physical trends on different levels, including physiological, hormonal, and biochemical processes. For example, your body has fat-burning enzymes that increase the rate and amount of fat broken down. These increase with consistent and higher levels of cardiovascular exercise. The stress of increased workouts over time causes the body to adapt and become better at burning fat.

JUST BURN IT!

When I was a child, my grandparents lived on a rural road that didn't have a garbage pickup service. To get rid of the garbage, my grandfather had an old steel barrel that we threw all the garbage into. Then he would burn it until only a few inches of ash remained at the bottom. As kids, this was a game to us. We would squirt lighter fluid on the fire, and it would cause larger flames to burn the garbage faster.

Your fat-burning enzymes act like lighter fluid in burning the fat faster and leaving only CO_2 and H_2O (instead of ashes). The levels of these hormones go up or down based on our activity levels over time. This means we can build fat-burning momentum through increased enzymes, which can be built and maintained.

FEELINGS OF WELL-BEING

A sense of well-being is not physiological or as easily defined or proven. Rather, it is emotional and psychological in nature. It is also somewhat subjective, meaning it is influenced by a person's thoughts, ideas, and tendencies. Even so, well-being is a real sensation we can feel.

When we exercise, we can increase our sense of well-being. Physiologically, this is caused as the body releases endorphins, which are feel-good chemicals in our brains. I'm sure you have heard the term *runners high*; this is a state in which the body produces a large amount of endorphins, and the runner experiences a natural high. Unfortunately, I don't think I have ever run long enough to get there!

There is also what I will call a "physical prowess" that results from the confidence that comes with increased strength, balance, and body control. These physiological changes of increased strength and body control make you feel enhanced physical confidence and safety.

YOUR NERVES ACTUALLY FUNCTION BETTER

Another physiological change that takes place as you eat right and work out is increased nerve innervation. The easiest way to explain this is if you have ever had a cast on your hand or foot. As a child, I broke my thumb. When the cast came off, my skin had less feeling, and I couldn't move my hand quickly or in a coordinated way. With use, all those things came back. In a sense, my nerves were "asleep" from not being used, but they were awakened with use.

When you exercise, you often see a rapid increase in strength, which is caused first by increased nerve activity from increased exercise. Building physical muscle is a longer process. In addition to increased strength, there will also be increased balance, coordination, and reaction time.

BUILD KINESTHETIC AWARENESS

A rough definition of *kinesthetic awareness* is your body's awareness in relation to space and objects. This sense allows us to navigate physical obstacles and situations. Exercise and activity increase this awareness. Increasing kinesthetic awareness can be the difference of tripping over something or bumping your head on something instead of ducking underneath it. When we watch athletes gracefully dodging, throwing, and catching, we are seeing highly developed kinesthetic awareness. While our goal is not to make the NBA or NFL, we can greatly increase our confidence and how we feel by increasing this ability through physical activity.

TRENDING

Our physical state and abilities are either trending in a positive or negative direction. When we deliberately focus our energies to make sure our momentum is headed in the right direction, we will make consistent progress. We must first stop negative trends and then work to get them going in the right direction. Along the way, if momentum is slowed, stopped, or even reversed, we must apply sufficient energy and force to get things going in the right direction again.

MAKE COMEBACKS FROM SETBACKS

I got frustrated after I pulled my back and toe muscles because my exercise levels decreased, my eating increased, and I gained some of the lost weight back. I was feeling fat again. So, I started my regular workouts again and abstained from meat for two weeks. Then one day after a hike, I looked in the mirror and noticed that I looked and felt different. I felt thinner and more muscular; something had shifted. Though it wasn't a huge physical change, (maybe two to three pounds lost since reengaging), something had shifted in how I felt. I felt good. I felt strong. I felt like I was on the right path again and moving forward. The momentum had changed, and I felt like I was trending in the right direction again.

Bottom line: Stop negative momentum and fight to maintain gains. Always reengage to build positive momentum when needed.

WEIGHT LOSS AS PROCESSES OR EVENT?

Most people treat weight loss as an event and that is why they end up fatter after their weight loss than before. On April 1, they look in the mirror and want to lose twenty pounds before summer so they will look good on the beach. They do unhealthy or unsustainable things to lose the weight and reach their goal. Let's say they lose twenty pounds by July; they completed their weight-loss event. But by August 1, they've gained back five to six pounds, and by Christmas, they weigh ten pounds more than when they started. The weight-loss event was successful, but the process failed in the long run.

If these same people focused on our three goals of building muscle, burning fat, and eating right, the results would be slower but longer lasting. They may have only lost ten of the twenty pounds by July 1, but by August 1, they'd have lost fifteen pounds, and by September 1, all twenty. The difference is that by Christmas, they'd have lost ten more pounds—a full thirty—and could keep it off.

EMBRACE THE PROCESS AND JOURNEY

You have spent your life becoming who you are physically today. I was deliberate about being strong and healthy as a teen and young adult, but my processes grew in an unhealthy direction as I decreased activity and made too many bad food choices over time. Life stage changes, like taking on responsibility for a wife and four children, bills, and work pushed my health habits in the wrong direction. I had to choose to stop the negative momentum and build positive momentum instead (and keep it going).

BIG IDEAS

Once you get things moving, momentum is built, which makes
our efforts easier and our new habits last longer.

You can build psychological and physiological momentum
to trend in the desired direction.

Physical confidence grows as your body strengthens
and your balance and coordination increases.

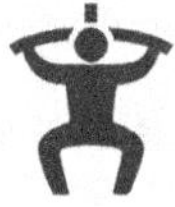

ACTION STEPS

Purposely build psychological momentum. Increase exposure
to positive people and influences while you minimize contact
with negative people and influences.

Embrace a new level of confidence.

Commit to exercise/be active three to six days a week every week.

FIGHT THE AGING PROCESS

The key to the future in an aging society is not found in increasing just our life span; we need to increase our health span at the same time.
—Chuck Norris[45]

As I started my health journey, I realized aging was magnifying the effects of my bad choices and body neglect. For the first time in my life, it was time to rally against aging. I had to shift from thinking, "Yeah, great, another thing to battle" to going into attack mode. Sometimes the fight chooses you; sometimes you choose the fight. The easiest way to lose a fight is to not fight back.

Whether you like it or not, age affects everybody. But here is the good news: behavior can affect the rate at which your body ages. I saw this clearly as I observed several men in their early sixties who were having trouble walking while other men in their seventies and eighties were active and still had a bounce in their step. The men in their sixties were painful examples of how age plus deterioration from lack of exercise and poor nutrition can literally destroy the body. In contrast, the men in their eighties were a testament to how physical activity and a healthy diet can keep you vibrant much longer.

So, what's going on? As we age, hormonal change, decreased physical activity, and reduced recovery rates all affect our physical vibrancy. We can't eliminate these age-related changes, but we can slow them down or reverse them if we alter our diet, sleep, and activity.

HORMONAL CHANGES

Men's testosterone and women's estrogen levels decrease with age. Hormonal changes can result in muscle loss and increased body fat. As discussed, both are bad for our metabolism. We've all seen radio and TV ads for products to increase testosterone. At first, I thought these were over-the-top ads that didn't apply to most men. But as I personally experienced a decrease in energy levels and an increase in fat storage, I saw why men would purchase these products. I don't have confidence that they work, but I get why you would want them to work.

WOMEN AND ESTROGEN

In women, estrogen levels change as does the overall balance of hormones. While these changes are part of maturing and going through menopause, the impact, such as decreased muscle and increased fat stores, can still be detrimental. The good news is these changes can be greatly affected by nutrition and exercise.[46] Medical intervention through hormone replacement is both a personal and medical decision that should be worked through with a doctor, but even when this approach is taken, diet and exercise are still major factors in a woman's well-being.

DECREASED PHYSICAL ACTIVITY MAKES MUSCLES SHRINK

With age, most people decrease their participation in recreational sports and exercise activities. This decrease can be more deleterious for wellness than hormonal decreases. Whether it's hectic schedules, work and family responsibilities, or less passion for physical activity, less movement is the general trend as we age. With less stress on our muscles through use and impact, muscles weaken and decrease, decreasing our rate of calorie burn and increasing fat storage. Muscle tightness, increased joint pain, and decreased endurance usually result. While exercise is medicine, leading to physical improvement, decreased activity leads to physical deterioration over time.

DECREASED RECOVERY RATES

With decreased hormonal levels, less efficient nutrient absorption, and other physiological changes, our bodies take longer to recover from exercise as we age. This causes us to either work out less intensely or need longer recovery times. We need to be conscious of our body and how much nutrition and rest we need to be able to exercise at desired levels.

Intentional modifications in nutrition, such as sufficient water, protein, calories, vitamins, and minerals, can powerfully affect how fast we recover and how hard our next workout can be.

DIABETES 101

Until someone has to deal with diabetes personally, most will not seek to understand what it is and how it can be avoided, reversed, or treated. Diabetes is caused by a person's body either becoming resistant to insulin or having a lack of insulin. Type 1 diabetes is when someone's pancreas does not produce sufficient insulin, which means they must take insulin shots. Onset is most common in young people. Type 2 diabetes usually occurs as people get older and fatter. As the body gains fat, it becomes resistant to absorbing blood glucose and then to insulin itself. Over time, the body produces more and more insulin and becomes more and more resistant to it.

Insulin is a storage hormone released when blood sugar goes up from eating. It pushes some of the sugar (glucose) from the food into muscles, stores some as glycogen (a concentrated form of sugar) in the muscles and liver, and then stores the rest as fat. Basically, it pushes sugars somewhere in the body besides the bloodstream. In people with diabetes, excess blood sugar damages and ages the body and then gets stored as fat. If someone is borderline or low-level diabetic, losing twenty pounds or so of fat will often push them out of the pre- or early diabetic state.

The fatter a person gets, the more likely they are to become diabetic, with additional fat causing diabetes to progressively worsen over time and making it easier and easier to keep packing on unwanted weight. I can still hear Dr. DeMeersman, from grad school at Columbia, calling it *diabesiosity*, meaning weight gain and diabetes feed each other. Basically, uncontrolled diabetes will make you obese and/or obesity will make you diabetic, and they will both create a cycle that will age and destroy your organs. Kind of bleak, but it is what it is.

Increasing muscle, decreasing body fat, increasing exercise, and improving nutrition can prevent onset and decrease or reverse diabetic trends, thereby protecting your kidneys, eyes, heart, brain, and circulatory system. Such measures, which were part of our ancestors' lifestyle, must now be implemented through purposeful food choice and planned exercise.

HEALTH IS OUR NORMAL STATE

As I just said, physical activity and eating naturally have been normal activities throughout the history of man. Industrialization, mechanization of work, modern travel, and the proliferation of manufactured food not only contribute to an unnatural lifestyle but can also cause our bodies to age faster.

LIVE LONGER AND HEALTHIER

If you ask me how long I want to live, I have two responses. The short answer is, I want to live long. But, if I had a choice of living long (say over one hundred years old) but not feeling good for the last thirty years or living to be seventy-five but feeling good my entire life, I would take fewer years feeling good. But no matter how long we live, we should seek to live a long and healthy life.

AGE/WEIGHT/ENERGY EQUATION

People don't die of old age; they die of neglect. –JACK LALANNE[47]

When it comes to our physical bodies, our age, physical weight, and daily energy levels are intertwined. How many times have you heard people say of rambunctious children playing, "I wish I had all that energy"? Children seem to have endless energy and can eat anything; this is directly connected to their age. For me, I was somewhat idealistic and delusional in thinking I would always have endless energy, even though I knew better.

EXPERIENCING WHAT I DIDN'T WANT

Unfortunately, I spent ten years learning through experience how age affects the body. I felt a shift around forty, another one at forty-five, and something different again at fifty. My metabolism slowed and my muscle tone and daily energy decreased. I learned that if you don't fight against aging, things progress more quickly.

We must combat the momentum of deterioration in muscle, strength, and endurance, which takes time and focus. My last decade started with four small children and finished with three teens and a preteen. A major career shift and other changes brought stress and difficulty. Even without added stress, these changes in our body just happen. However, if we passively accept the changes, then they happen even faster and more dramatically.

WEIGHT MAINTENANCE CAN BE DECEIVING

If you are maintaining your current bodyweight, that is better than gaining weight (excess fat), but it can be deceiving. Let me explain. If ten years goes by and each year you lose one pound of muscle from age or decreased activity and you gain just one pound of fat, then over the decade you will have lost ten pounds of muscle and gained ten pounds of fat while weighing the same amount. Imagine this starts at eighteen. At twenty-eight, you would be proud of weighing the same as high school graduation. If the trend continues for the next decade, at your twentieth reunion, you could smile and say, "I haven't gained a pound since graduation!" The reality is, however, you have twenty pounds less muscle and twenty pounds more fat. This sets the stage to go into your forties and fifties ready to put on weight.

MUSCLE VS. FAT WEIGHT

As we talk about weight, keep a simple principle in mind. Adding muscle and muscle weight is good and healthy. Adding excessive fat and fat weight is physically unhealthy. So, for instance, if a person is lifting weights and doing cardio and gains five pounds of muscle but loses five pounds of fat over six months, they will weigh the same but feel and look much better. Remember, our goal is to build more muscle and lose excess fat. Since most people are carrying excess fat, even when they gain muscle, overall, there will be a net weight loss.

PAIN OF CHANGE OR PAIN OF STAYING THE SAME

Most people hate change as it is disruptive and often painful. It has often been said that people won't change until the pain of staying the same is greater than the pain of change. I hit that point; the pain of maintaining my course became unbearable. I knew I was playing a losing game in several areas of my life, including my bodyweight. My problems had grown over time until I hated several paths I was on. Weight was one facet of life I could and did change.

SHOULD OR MUST?

I reached a breaking point; I hated the condition of my health. I switched from "I should live differently" to "I must live differently." I no longer had another option. When the pain of staying the same became unbearable, I had to either make significant changes or just give up. My path became clear. For too long, I took my weight gain as a joke, but I wasn't laughing anymore.

MY BODY'S RESPONSE TO FOOD CHANGED

If I eat the same exact food now that I used to eat, I will now gain weight. I don't even have to eat more. If I simply eat the same type and amount of foods I used to eat, instead of maintaining the same weight, I get fatter.

For example, this may sound funny, but I can almost gauge my weight loss or gain by whether or not I put sugar in my coffee. This is something fairly recent. For some reason, when I drink black coffee, I tend to lose weight, but if I drink coffee with milk and sugar, I tend to gain weight. Something changed in my body where it doesn't process sugar as well as it used to. Now, for the first time in my life, adding a little sugar to my diet is enough to put on weight. With age and hormonal changes, a couple of teaspoons of sugar is enough to trigger increased insulin production and fat storage.

MORE DILIGENT WITH EATING

I didn't mean to gain weight, it happened by snackcident.[48]

Honestly, I was blessed with a good metabolism. So, until my mid-forties, I was able to eat just about anything I wanted as long as I was reasonably active. But now, I must be more careful and diligent with my food choices and amounts. In fact, I tell people that, at times, the most important exercise we can do is the push-away. After the second plate of food, push away from the table. I target the second plate because most don't want to hear about being overly strict.

Basically, if I am consistently making the right food choices and working out properly, I will be fine. I do snack and occasionally will eat just about anything in limited amounts. For instance, if I eat well all week and have a fudge brownie sundae with my kids over the weekend, I'm not stressing about it, especially if I am in a maintenance stage. When I was focused on fat burning, I would stay away from sweet treats entirely.

You can't totally stop the aging process, but your food choice and activity level can definitely slow it down and reverse the results of bad habits or neglect.

BIG IDEAS

Your body changes with age.

Decreased activity and poor food choices will age you faster.

You can slow down and reverse age-related physical changes through increased activity and good food choices.

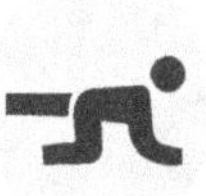

ACTION STEPS

Read articles, books, and blogs (by reputable people) on how the body works and how to fight the aging process.

Discipline yourself to exercise. One of my goals is not to go two days without going to the gym or exercising in some way because two days easily turns into three or four.

Purposely choose foods with a variety of health benefits (i.e., foods to fight high cholesterol, promote a healthy brain or heart, etc.).

MANAGE TIME

We all get 24 hours a day . . . It's up to us as to what we do with those twenty-four hours.

—Sam Huff [49]

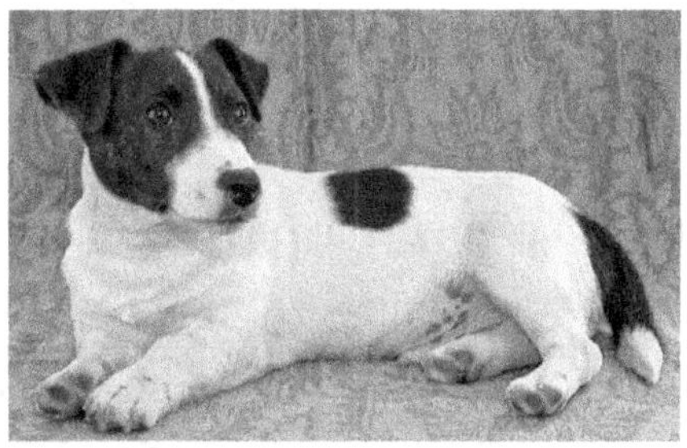

One factor leading to my success may not seem like it has anything to do with weight loss, but it was key: time management. Most who know me would consider me one of the busiest people they know. This means I have many legitimate reasons to skip workouts, slack off, and not eat right. But my health became a greater priority and then an absolute top priority for the last two months of reaching my goal. When I scheduled my days and better managed my time, the whole world saw the results. This concept was something I had learned before, but this recent experience definitely took it to a new level.

LESSONS LEARNED FROM A DOG

I learned an unexpected lesson when I got a new puppy. My kids and I wanted a dog. One of our daughters named Luther several years before we got him. Every once in a while, we would sit at the kitchen table and talk about Luther before he was ours.

I like to take my daughters on Daddy dates. On one of those dates, we drove past a place with a big sign that said puppies, and we went in to see them. I am fairly familiar with dogs but wasn't familiar with the particular breed. They were small dogs with a big dog attitude: Irish Jack Russel Terriers—and they were from Ireland.

I asked about them and learned they are related to the American Jack Russel Terrier but are shorter, more muscular, and more mellow in temperament. We played, and I asked questions. The breeder told me they were fifteen hundred dollars. I smiled because I didn't have fifteen dollars for a dog, never mind fifteen hundred. Between two litters, we met fourteen to fifteen dogs total, but one was our favorite.

Over the next couple of months, we visited occasionally. Then, the funniest thing happened. Over time every other dog was bought, except our favorite. The breeder had taken a liking to my daughter and me and told us she wanted to give us the dog. Luther was ours. Each morning, I spent about an hour walking and training Luther. We added another two to three walks to the day, with the last one right before bed.

MY LIFE WAS BUSY

This was in 2011. Our family was in debt following the housing bubble burst. I suffered a pay cut at my full-time job, and the thirty to forty speaking engagements I booked annually at different churches all but disappeared, along with the income they brought. Lastly, I ran a nonprofit where donations decreased by about 90 percent. Not a good time!

We had a house with a mortgage. With four children between ages three and seven, my wife had stopped working to take care of them. I was working multiple jobs, didn't have enough money, and struggled to have time with my wife and kids. I didn't have enough time to exercise, rest, or have fun. But somehow, I was able to find one hour every morning (and multiple other times a day) for Luther.

Most of us say we are too busy to take care of our body. I'd like to share what I learned from Luther, in case it inspires you to needed action: I had time for what was important.

For some reason, this puppy was able to command over one hour of my time *every* day. If you asked me the week before I got the dog if I had any extra time, I would have said no. But out of nowhere, I had an extra hour each day. The reality was that I had time for whatever I deemed important. Here are some practical steps that can help us:

1. **Make a choice:** You have to make a choice to change your routine or schedule. Without solid determination, you will simply follow your normal patterns. Most of the losing-weight process happens in your mind.

2. **Commit the time:** If I could commit time to a dog's well-being, why couldn't I commit time to my own well-being? For successful weight loss, you must commit time to exercise and food preparation. You do have time for food preparation and exercise—*if* you make these activities nonnegotiable.

I think the greatest factor in reaching my goal weight was committing to at least thirty minutes a day for fifty-one days on the elliptical. On top of that, I would do fifteen to twenty minutes of resistance training six days a week after I finished the elliptical. This effort made me more focused on food choice and timing. One good choice led to another; it was a chain reaction of fat-burning momentum. My time commitment to the gym changed everything.

ALLOW THE BENEFITS TO MOTIVATE YOU

Let every healthy meal and exercise session motivate you. Allow yourself to feel good about your efforts and to enjoy the increased health you experience. Ongoing motivation is needed for lasting change to stick. Take the time to be proud of your effort and positive changes. You are not only getting healthier, but you are also growing as a person. You are doing something noble that affects the quality of your life. Being healthier benefits family and friends because they want us to be healthy. It even benefits society as a whole as a healthier person tends to be happier and more productive than average.

PLANNING REST AND RECUPERATION

Rest when you're weary. Refresh and renew yourself, your body, your mind, your spirit. Then get back to work. –RALPH MARSTON[50]

Let's talk about doing nothing. For some people, this comes easily. Frequent naps, going to bed early, even staying in bed all day and all night is no problem. Not so much for me. I am pretty bad at resting. I don't even like sitting still. Always on the move, I'm working, writing, traveling, doing, doing, doing. The problem is, our bodies need rest to counterbalance the motion.

When we talk about planning, our mind's natural flow usually goes to planning what to do, like finishing tasks or achieving goals. But when it comes to being healthy, one of the most important factors is rest and recuperation. As I age, rest has become more of a nonnegotiable, but with all my passions and responsibilities, I still have to fight to rest properly.

OUR CULTURE FIGHTS TIMES OF REST

We live in the busiest culture in the history of the world. The average person in America is overbooked. We work hard, run up credit cards, and take out loans that control our lives. We train our children to be super active, which makes parents super busy. Our phones buzz and ring with texts, calls, and e-mails so that we are constantly on, whether it's work or family related. We go to bed later and wake up earlier, and most of us don't get enough rest. But rest has many benefits we must keep in mind.

BETTER OVERALL HEALTH

Our body needs rest. We are not made to work nonstop, never giving our body time to rejuvenate. Sufficient sleep is basic to health. The recommended amount of daily sleep for adults aged eighteen to sixty is seven or more hours.[51] While sleeping, our mind and body relax. Our heart rate and blood pressure go down. Our mind can shut down instead of racing between responsibilities, life issues, and personal conflicts. Like our body, our minds need rest. During stressful times, including weight loss, your body may require additional sleep at night or naps when possible.

REST IS RECUPERATIVE

Our bodies are constantly rebuilding on a cellular level. This takes place during sleep. Insufficient sleep means our body will not rebuild itself to an optimal level. This includes muscles. Even if decreased rest doesn't lead to sickness, it will result in performing at a lower level with increased fatigue and decreased health.

Muscle strains, joint sprains, and muscle pain all heal during sleep. Insufficient rest will hinder the recuperation processes. When I sprained my spine, the only explanation was that my body was tight from too much stress and worn down from insufficient rest. Thus, merely twisting to get out of the car sprained the ligaments on my spine.

While it's hard to believe the worst injury of my life happened by getting out of my car, I experienced it and know it's true. I did some crazy things in my life (eight years of football, martial arts on concrete floors and in backyards, mosh pits, barroom brawls, mountain bike crashes, four wheeling, squatting over six hundred pounds, deadlifting over four hundred pounds, power cleans, and kettlebells), but, ironically, insufficient rest contributed to the ultimate injury. I was totally incapacitated for months by getting out of my car to get my oil changed. Stress and fatigue are real and detrimental to your health without sufficient rest.

REST HELPS EMOTIONAL HEALTH

Fatigue has caused many problems in my life. I've experienced physical, emotional, and relational problems due to a lack of rest. You may be thinking, *What do you mean?* When I am tired, I have less patience and am more sarcastic and short-tempered. Not good for my marriage, my kids, or any relationship, work or social.

Physical fatigue can also cause mental fatigue, resulting in loss of happiness, discouragement, and lack of motivation. Unhealthy emotions often lead to overeating. Increased relational conflict and relational distress can also lead to emotional eating. By not resting sufficiently, we tend to overeat. I'm often faced with the choice of eating more to regain focus and power through or stopping work, but deadlines and upcoming or overdue bills drive me to eat and keep going.

THE POWER OF NAPS

The term *power nap* refers to a short nap that rejuvenates or gives a person power. It's aptly named because it can stop the trend toward fatigue and rejuvenate you physically and mentally.

I don't seem to have the ability to take a fifteen-minute power nap, but I have taken one- to two-hour naps that help me be a better human. I joke that, over the years, my wife has told me several times to go take a nap. Yes, dear.

PLANNED RECUPERATION

In addition to sleeping, you should plan times of physical rest from exercise. This can mean resting a day or two between resistance exercise sessions or building rest days into your running schedule. In your weight-loss efforts, you will increase the stress on your body, which may require increased rest. Remember, rest is when your body is growing stronger.

Rest and recuperation can also help you avoid and overcome injury. Pain and injury are your body's way of letting you know you are either doing too much or did something that caused harm. Exercise, by definition, places stress on your body. Rest gives your body needed time and space to build health.

YOU HAVE TIME FOR WHAT MATTERS TO YOU

People don't like to hear it, but you do have time for the things that matter most to you. We all have the same twenty-four hours, and we choose how to manage them. If you discipline yourself to stick to and execute your plans, you will reach your goal, but you have to put in the work.

BIG IDEAS

We must plan times of rest to be healthy.

Rest and recuperation are needed both physically and emotionally.

Excessive hunger or fatigue is your body telling you to
slow down or stop and rest.

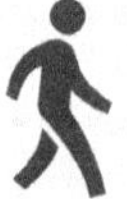

ACTION STEPS

Plan a reasonable amount of work or activity in your schedule.

Schedule times of rest, vacation, or a day off periodically.

Purposely take naps or have quiet times alone to decompress.

MANAGE STRESS

Warning: Chocolate makes your clothes shrink.[52]

Managing stress was key to my weight loss. People often tell me that I never seem stressed or act stressed. I may look calm on the outside, but when stressed, I tend to eat excessively and make bad food choices. If you go to the gym and burn five hundred calories and then eat five hundred extra calories to manage stress, you just erased the benefit of your hard work.

OVEREATING BECAUSE OF STRESS AND EMOTIONS

Our fast-paced and overbooked lives often lead to excessive stress, which can push us to bad food choices and overeating. In many seasons of my life, I ate two meals a day in my car, working and going from place to place, eating along the way. Translated, this means I ate two fast-food meals a day. My fast pace led to the exact opposite of eating right; I ate the wrong foods at the wrong time.

OVERSCHEDULING CAUSES UNHEALTHY PHYSICAL RESPONSES

Stress causes our bodies to release excessive adrenaline, resulting in a short-term energy burst. This is followed by an energy drop that we often address with a nice dose of junk food. Salt, sugar, and fat can give us a short boost, but it is the worst thing we can do if we want to reach or maintain a healthy weight.

DRAMA

Unfortunately, our lives are also often filled with problems, conflicts, and drama of all sorts. This is when chocolate screams the loudest to me. Cookies call to me too. Just kidding, sort of. Maybe it's my flesh crying out for the chocolate, but I know something is telling me to eat it.

RELATIONSHIPS AND EMOTIONAL EATING

Whether we like it or not, relationships cause stress, and we often self-medicate with food. After a disagreement or when feeling lonely, I have soothed with a bowl of ice cream. Many times, after working late and getting home to my sleeping wife and kids, I look to a bowl of ice cream to fill the gap where human connection should be. But emotional eating adds up. My solution: I don't even buy ice cream now. If I don't plan proactively, it will be me and the bowl of ice cream on the couch watching *Animal Planet*.

UNFINISHED TASKS AND FAMILY MANAGEMENT

Marriage has taught me that we are different than our spouse. For instance, after a long day of dealing with issues and drama, I want to end my day quietly, not thinking of unfinished tasks, needs, or problems. My wife is the exact opposite. At the end of the day, she likes to unload any problems, conflicts, or unfinished tasks because after venting, she feels peaceful and can go to sleep.

Imagine this scenario: Right before going to bed, I am quiet and peaceful. Then my wife rattles off a list of everything wrong with the house, the kids, the bills, and anything else broken on Planet Earth. After she lets it go, she can roll over and go to sleep as I lie awake thinking of ways to fix the twenty-seven problems just listed. Too many times, this leaves me wide awake and wanting a glass of milk and cookies to deal with the stress and relax to go to sleep.

Your story is different, but it is helpful to understand what triggers you to overeat. Then you can work these things out. To meet my wife's concerns, I had to make sure I spoke with her at other times to address the family's needs. I also needed to ask her not to unload in a way that would keep me up and lead me to overeat. This is weight loss in the real world.

If I don't properly address these dynamics and unmet family needs, I can start to feel overwhelmed and lonely because my wife is asleep, and I'm left dealing with these problems. The ice cream starts calling my name.

The reality is, ice cream works—temporarily. It soothes and takes my focus off the problems. If this happens twice a week for a year (with a bowl of ice cream at two hundred fifty calories), it adds up to twenty-six thousand calories or about seven-and-a-half pounds of fat in just one year. That's over twenty pounds of fat in just three years. Therefore, I had to learn to manage these real-life dynamics to avoid packing on more weight.

DEFEATING STRESS AND NEGATIVE EMOTIONS

When working toward a healthy body weight, you must minimize and navigate stress. Here are a few steps to get stress under control:

1. Make a list of all activities that eat up your time. Once you see all you are doing, cross off and stop doing things that waste time and don't help you make life progress.

2. Prioritize activities: List what is most important to you and focus your time and energy on those things. When you get to a point of fatigue, stop and pick it up again the next day.

3. Eat healthy snacks: Take time to buy and prepare nutritional snacks so that when you are stressed out you will have needed nutrition—instead of empty calories—on hand. In addition to raw fruits/vegetables, I often eat egg whites, almonds, or high-fiber Ezekiel muffins.

COMBATTING THE EXTREMES

The extremes of overtired and overstressed lead us to turn to food to numb and cope. The reality is, if we get to a certain point of distress, we will overeat, overcaffeinate, and over rely on junk food. So how do we combat extreme lows?

EAT REGULARLY

When we eat three basic meals and healthy snacks, several things are achieved. First, we supply the body with essential nutrients. This keeps us feeling better due to sufficient caloric intake. Having sufficient energy also keeps our emotions healthier, so we are less stressed out, which helps us feel less grumpy and argumentative—and those negative states both sap energy.

With regular meals, our blood sugar levels also stay in a healthier zone, which decreases fatigue, cravings, and extreme hunger.

GET SUGAR FROM FRUITS AND VEGETABLES

Many people don't realize that fruits and vegetables have simple sugars in them. When we are crashing and craving junk, it is because of low blood sugar. Instead of that cookie or chocolate bar, a handful of trail mix with dried fruits and nuts can give you the boost you need. But with the added fiber, protein, and fat of nuts, you enjoy a slower and more gradual increase in blood sugar and avoid the spikes and dips junk food gives.

I often pack an apple, banana, and orange for my day and eat them whether or not I want them between meals or after dinner. In this way, I head off blood sugar crashes that will tempt me toward junk. I also learned that drinking a glass of water can give me more enduring energy through proper hydration than that next coffee and candy bar because that's what I needed.

FIGHTING THROUGH DISCOURAGEMENT

When I committed to losing thirty-five pounds and exercised that first week, I gained three pounds. What? Remember, my plan was to lose one pound per week. How did I gain three? That was discouraging, but I persisted. I'm so glad I did.

Life drama also makes losing and keeping weight off more difficult. Crisis and conflict can consume us, drain us, and cause us to retreat from the fight for weight loss. We must fight and battle through the distractions that pull us away and instead stay true to the discipline of weight loss.

It's not a matter of *if* stress and drama will hit us; it's a matter of *when*. Personal conflicts cause pain, drain us, and make things overly complicated. That's when we must choose: either turn to food as our comfort medicine and anti-stressor and fall into numbing out with TV or social media or turn to exercise to burn off the stress and bring us back to peace and focus.

THE FEAR OF FAILURE

Any time you attempt something big in life, you will have to face and overcome doubt and even fear. Past failures can magnify these emotions. I was carrying unwanted fat because my previous efforts had either failed or, after success, I didn't maintain discipline, so I regained unwanted fat. Achieving and maintaining positive mind space and attitude are key to ongoing success.

STAYING FOCUSED IN THE STRESS

We must stay focused on our dream. For me, my ongoing destination is 190 pounds. Even when I face stress, roadblocks, and detours, or I simply mess up, I must refocus on my vision. My goal of 190 steers my food choices and activities. When I am wrestling with doubt or fear of failure, my destination determines my actions. It doesn't matter what I feel or what others say, I know my goal. It's funny, but many times, people told me I didn't need to lose more weight, but if I listened to those voices, I would be distracted from my focus.

I've learned not to be emotional about my food choices. I simply eat food that is good for me. I'm not moved by whether or not I want to exercise; I simply exercise. Feelings are secondary issues when I am committed to my goals. We do this all the time with other things; we can do it with food and exercise also. Think about it: How many school assignments did you do that you didn't feel like doing? How many personal and job-related tasks do you do each day that you don't necessarily want to do or maybe even dislike doing? I've done thousands of loads of laundry, but I never wanted to do a single one—same for doing the dishes. As a husband and father, I do things every day and often all day that I don't have a desire to do, even things I dislike. It's called life. I can apply this principle to my fat-loss efforts, too: do the right thing whether you are feeling it or not.

Yes, the struggle is real, but you can do it. Set the goal. Don't be deterred by fear, stress, or doubt. Set your eyes on your goal and don't stop going until you get there.

BIG IDEAS

List your activities and tasks and then prioritize them
to focus on the most important ones. This will reduce stress.

Crisis, conflict, and discouragement are part of life and must be
managed and pushed through.

Eat consistent meals and snacks to supply sufficient nutrition
and resist the temptation of junk food.

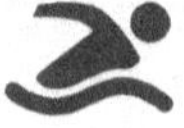

ACTION STEPS

Purposely manage your stress by taking breaks to decompress.

After you make a list of priorities, schedule time blocks
for your major priorities.

Pack healthy snacks that you plan to eat at stressful or predetermined times. For example, while writing this book, I would often work later in the night so I would bring my bag of "rabbit food" (three carrots, three stalks of celery, and half a cucumber chopped in pieces) and eat it from eight to ten instead of a candy bar and soda.

MOVE TO HEAL

Movement is a medicine for creating change in a person's physical, emotional, and mental states. –CAROL WELCH-BARIL [53]

One of my key transitional moments occurred when I returned to the gym after I sprained my spine. Working out again helped me regain a sense of control over my body and my life. Fear, self-pity, and helplessness were replaced with hope and a positive attitude.

Movement promotes health, functions as preventative medicine, has psychological benefits, and helps heal injuries. It can also reverse and correct degenerative processes set in motion by inactivity and poor eating habits.

WHAT YOU GAIN FROM LOSING

Being healthy isn't about the weight you lose, it's about the life you gain. [54]

Losing fat, especially through eating well and exercising, helps you gain many things. Addition by subtraction? Let's take a look at some of the physiological and emotional wins.

Increased Energy

If I had a dollar for every time I heard someone say, "I'm tired," I'd be a rich man. Healthy weight loss adds energy while simultaneously decreasing energy drain. Imagine walking around with a forty-pound backpack all day long, every day. That's exactly what I was doing; I was carrying around forty extra pounds for no good reason.

Increased Heart Health and Strength

During the weight-loss process, when done gradually with exercise, two things happen to your heart. First your heart grows stronger due to increased exercise. Your heart is a muscle, so when you are walking, jogging, or on the treadmill, it's not only your leg muscles getting stronger, but your heart is getting stronger also. With increased fitness, you will notice your resting pulse (how many times your heart beats per minute) decreases.

Increased heart strength causes the heart to pump more blood with each beat, requiring less beats per minute to pump either the same or even more blood to your body. Do the math. If your heart rate decreased from eighty to seventy beats per minute, that's six hundred fewer beats in an hour and 7,200 less beats per day or 50,400 less beats per week.

With less fat, the heart has less blood to pump. Since one pound of fat has one mile of capillaries, with every pound of fat you lose,[55] your heart has to pump less blood to supply the body with what it needs. Imagine if everywhere you walked all day was uphill. How tired would you be at the end of the day? That's the condition your heart is under when you are carrying unnecessary fat. It has to work harder every time it beats.

Increased Muscle

Resistance training increases muscle size and strength, making many tasks easier. Picking up your child or doing yard work won't require as much exertion when your muscle mass increases. And you'll have fewer injuries and less pain in your back or joints. As I got a little older and stopped lifting weights, I felt pain in my joints. After I began lifting weights and using resistance machines again, the pain went away. Stronger muscles provide greater support to the joints and also absorb the shock of walking, jogging, and moving (instead of our bones and joints).

Increased HDL (Good Cholesterol)

When we talk about high cholesterol, we are referring to bad cholesterol. This is low-density lipoprotein (LDL), which is the cholesterol that sticks to your blood vessels and causes blockages leading to heart attacks or strokes. High-density lipoproteins (HDL) is the good kind of cholesterol. It is hard cholesterol that scrapes away the LDL cholesterol in our blood vessels. HDL can be increased through eating healthier, especially high-fiber foods such as oatmeal, whole grains, and raw vegetables. Some alkaline substitutes for oatmeal include amaranth, kamut, spelt, rye, or quinoa flakes.[56] Resistance training is another way to increase HDL cholesterol,[57] which helps keep our blood vessels clear.

Emotional and Psychological Benefits

Gaining muscle can cause us to feel an increased sense of confidence and well-being. This results from a greater sense of body control, stability, and strength, which is both physical and psychological. We see increased confidence, even arrogance, in teen boys when their muscles start to develop and they feel the power of their stronger bodies. Though we don't have to become egomaniacs or flex in the mirror every time we pass, we should embrace the healthy sense of physical strength that results in greater physical confidence.

Another aspect in terms of confidence is feeling good about looking better. Who doesn't want to look better? For me, I don't know if looking better was my goal, but I sure don't want to look worse. When I went to the fifth-grade daddy/daughter dance with my daughter, I was given motivation as to what I don't want to look like.

Decreased Depression and Anxiety

The Mayo Clinic has determined that exercise can decrease depression and anxiety. Regular exercise may help ease depression and anxiety by doing the following:[58]

- Releasing feel-good endorphins, which are natural brain chemicals that can enhance your sense of well-being.
- Taking your mind off worries so you can get away from the cycle of negative thoughts that feed depression and anxiety.

Exercise has many psychological and emotional benefits, too. This same study found that regular exercise can help you:

- Gain confidence: Meeting exercise goals or challenges, even small ones, can boost your self-confidence. Getting in shape can also make you feel better about your appearance.
- Get more social interaction: Exercise and physical activity may give you the chance to meet or socialize with others.

Just exchanging a friendly smile or greeting as you walk around your neighborhood can help your mood.

- Cope in a healthy way: Doing something positive to manage depression or anxiety is a healthy coping strategy. Trying to feel better by drinking alcohol, dwelling on how you feel, or hoping depression or anxiety will go away on its own can lead to worsening symptoms.

Some research shows that physical activity such as regular walking—not just formal exercise programs—may help improve mood. Physical activity and exercise are not the same thing, but both are beneficial to your health.

Physical Activity: any activity that works your muscles and requires energy; this can include work or household chores or leisure activities.

Exercise: a planned, structured, and repetitive body movement done to improve or maintain physical fitness.

Doing thirty minutes or more of exercise a day for three to five days a week may significantly improve depression or anxiety symptoms. But smaller amounts of physical activity—as little as ten to fifteen minutes at a time—may make a difference.

Relational Benefits

You'll also notice relational benefits as you get in shape. First, confident people are more attractive. The way you carry yourself makes a difference in how people perceive and treat you. Right or wrong, that's usually the way it goes. While people have different criteria for physical appearance, they usually find a more fit and confident person more attractive. Being in better shape can also help performance in the bedroom. Added muscle and endurance can benefit both you and your partner, not only in performance and ability to satisfy your partner but also in increased desire.

EXERCISE TO OVERCOME INJURY

One of the unexpected obstacles to my weight loss was injury. Age and weaker muscles were factors. I used to be able to do anything without injury, yet within a year and a half, I had a laundry list of injuries, including lower back strain, pulled big toes, shoulder pain, neck spasms, and a sprained spine. I had to work through these pains while using exercise to heal and prevent further injury.

PAST INJURIES

Many of us have injuries or physical problems that limit us or eliminate certain activities. In high school, I broke my left big toe at the beginning of my senior basketball season. I didn't tell anyone because I wanted to play. I knew it was my last year of playing basketball, and I was fighting for a starting position. It healed crooked and is one of the reasons I don't jog because it throws off my gait, which causes other things to hurt. In college I had two major knee injuries in which I tore both ACLs and had to have them reconstructed. In graduate school, I used Rollerblades® a lot and used my right leg as my break leg, which caused damage to my right patellar tendon, resulting in tendonitis that is easily aggravated. Bottom line: I can't jog without causing all kinds of issues, so that's a limitation I have to work around. Many others I know have a bad back, flat feet, or unstable shoulders that cause limitations to the type or amount of activity they can do.

DO WHAT YOU CAN DO

While we all have certain limitations, there are many things we can do. Don't let what you can't do get in the way of what you can.

I can't jog, but I love hiking. You couldn't pay me to jog three miles, but one of my favorite things to do is my three-and-a-half-mile hike. I can also do low- or no-impact aerobic exercise, like bike riding, the elliptical, and swimming. I enjoy lifting weights and training with weight machines, cables, and kettlebells. Find and do what you can.

DISLIKES

Unfortunately, I hate jogging. In addition to my physical limitations, I simply don't like jogging. I find it difficult, boring, and even uncomfortable. I wish I did like jogging because, in my opinion, it is the simplest, most effective, and best bang for your buck in terms of time investment of any exercise. If you can jog twenty to thirty minutes three days a week, do it. You will burn fat, strengthen your heart, and see benefits from investing a relatively short amount of time.

INJURIES ALONG THE WAY

All the world is full of suffering. It is also full of overcoming.
—HELEN KELLER[59]

After I dropped the first ten pounds, I slipped on ice and came crashing down. As I was salting the sidewalk in front of my house, my feet flew from underneath me, and I crashed to the ground. My wife watched me fall and get up. Her eyes were the size of saucers as she asked me if I was okay. Yes, I hit hard, but I felt fine. I was not happy to fall, but everything seemed fine.

THREE HOURS LATER

I went on with my day with no problems. But as I was working from home that day, I printed a document on our home printer, and a paper fell on the ground. As I bent over to pick it up, I felt an excruciating pain in my lower back. Instantly, my back was frozen in pain, and I couldn't move. My back locked up. This was new to me and seemed to come out of nowhere.

FOUR DAYS LATER

Sunday morning came, and I was still in pain. When I sat for a while, I couldn't get up. Forget about exercising; I couldn't even stand up straight. When I walked, I looked like a broken old man.

It took about two weeks before I could do anything and then another two weeks of slowly building up to my full workout. I lost my momentum and a month of progress and weight loss. My goal of losing thirty-five pounds in thirty-five weeks was sidetracked. Yet, setbacks are part of life, and we must work within the limitations of reality and not get discouraged.

I PULLED MY TOE MUSCLE

Yes, it's possible to injure your toe muscle. I'm not sure how, but I pulled the muscle in my left big toe, and somehow, my toe was out of joint. After a couple of days of pain, I rubbed it and popped it back into place, but the tendons continued to hurt for a couple of weeks. Whenever I walked too much, they would burn with pain. Then a week or two later, I pulled the tendon in my right big toe. Most of you probably didn't even know you could pull a toe muscle. This was the first time in my life something like this happened. We have to deal with these things when they pop up. By the way, that meant no hiking (my favorite exercise) for a couple of months.

Once again, I had to modify workouts as I eliminated hiking, walking on a treadmill, and doing the elliptical. You, like me, will have to work around any injuries you experience. We can't let a temporary injury defeat us. Instead, modify your workouts to keep positive momentum going.

WHAT DO I DO WITH THIS?

"What do I do with this?" has become my go-to question in difficult situations. Life often blindsides us with difficult situations. I wanted to exercise and drop weight, yet I could barely move. I had to consider my situation and adjust.

DEALING WITH OBSTACLES

I went from cruising down the highway going seventy miles per hour to barely being able to walk. If I had been jogging, it would have been like running into a wall that wouldn't move. I'm sorry to say, but I am fairly confident you will also face obstacles on your road to weight loss. These may be physical or emotional obstacles, but you must learn to maneuver around them as they arise.

DEALING WITH INJURIES

I couldn't lift weights, stretch, or do any exercise at all. So, I dealt with the reality of being injured with the following steps.

First, I had to rest. Giving myself permission to rest was not easy because I don't like to rest. Resting makes me feel lazy, and from a practical sense, I knew I couldn't lose weight from resting. But reality mandated I rest.

Second, I had to go to the doctor. I'm one of those guys who doesn't take medicine or go to the doctor unless I have no other choice or need to please my wife. So, I went to the doctor for both of these reasons. I don't like doctors and didn't want to spend the money or take medicine. And, oh, yeah, my pride was also an issue; you know, I'm too strong and manly to be injured.

Last, I had to gradually return to exercise and build intensity over time. I had to use wisdom as I challenged myself to get better but was careful not to push myself too hard, which could prolong or increase my injury.

It took about a week before I could move sufficiently for things to fall back in place and two more weeks to work back to where I had been.

I could not let frustration and physical pain discourage me. I had to go through a tough season but stay committed to my goal. I had to take misfortune as a speed bump, not a roadblock. I had to cut back on food, and even though I couldn't exercise, I still lost two more pounds.

SPRAINING MY SPINE

I thought my first back injury was bad, but I had no idea of real pain until I sprained my spine. This injury became one of many opportunities I had to overcome injuries and setbacks. As I write about handling setbacks, know that I have lived it out myself. Injuries will come, so prepare to deal with them well.

One Friday morning, as I was getting out of my car to get my oil changed, I experienced shooting back pain across my lower back. My back spasmed, and I had trouble standing up. This continued every time I went from sitting to standing for the next three weeks.

These spasms lasted longer and were more excruciating than any pain I had ever experienced. Ice, physical therapy, and a chiropractor slowly helped over the next few weeks, but then I got to a standstill with my back, and everything else felt like it was deteriorating or falling apart.

My right hip started hurting. A tendon started clicking on the outside of my right knee, and I could feel my body deconditioning and becoming weaker. Terrible back spasms, increased joint pain, and decreased endurance were all starting to wear on me physically and emotionally.

BACK TO THE GYM

On day thirteen of spasms, I told my physical therapist and chiropractor that I wanted to go back to the gym for light workouts. Here is the workout I used:

- Walk on treadmill for five minutes
- Elliptical for five minutes
- Stretch ten minutes
- Light weight machines (e.g., twenty pounds on bench press machine)
- Five to ten minutes stretching

When I started going to the gym, something changed. Almost immediately I started feeling better, both physically and emotionally. My back spasms decreased. My hip felt better, and my knee stopped clicking. My overall energy also increased.

EXERCISE AS MEDICINE

Instinctively, I knew I needed to start back to exercising. I needed to feel better physically. Exhaustion was setting in because pain drains you. Pain is discouraging; the limitations my injury brought made me depressed.

I was also wrestling with the idea that some or all of my pain could be permanent, which discouraged me. I was reminded of this possibility every time I went from sitting to standing as I felt excruciating pain.

EXERCISE GAVE ME HOPE

Exercise gave me hope that I could return to a normal life. It restored a sense of control over my life. For the first time in my life, I couldn't stand up because of pain. Many more times when I stood up, I couldn't walk for several minutes. Being able to do basic exercise gave me hope that I could get better. With each exercise and each stretch, hope grew. I saw a path forward. Exercise helped more than anti-inflammatory meds and even muscle relaxers.

THE COMEBACK TRAIL

When injured, you have to make a comeback. If you do too much too soon, you will set yourself back. The more purposeful and systematic your rehabilitation is, the faster and more complete your return will likely be. Let's look at it in phases.

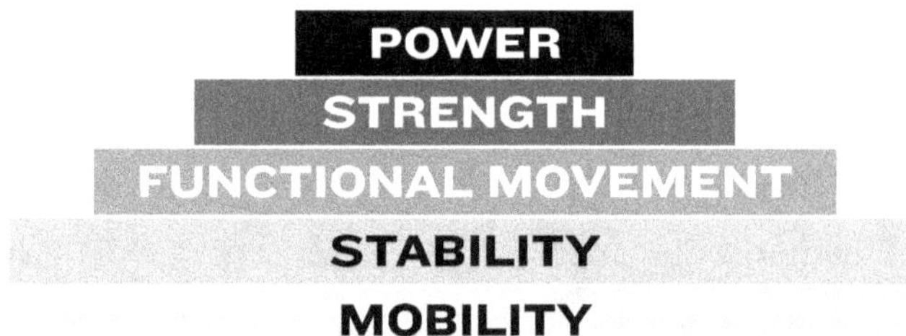

Mobility: I literally couldn't move. I had to break the pain-spasm cycle with ice, muscle relaxers, and then physical therapy and chiropractic care over weeks and months. As I gained mobility, the more I moved, the more I gained.

Stability: This required muscle-strengthening exercises for the entire body, with a focus on core muscles to support the injured area. In addition to core exercises, I used weight machines focusing on two sets of eight to ten exercises on all major muscle groups.

Functional Movement: Once I was more mobile and stable, I was able to add functional movements, like weight on machines, light dumbbells, barbells, and introductory HIIT exercises. If I felt pain in my back during these movements, I would stop, refocus on what I could do, and then progress back to them over time.

Strength: The next shift was regaining lost muscle from decreased activity. Basically, I was putting the overload principle to work, adding repetitions and then weight to different exercises over time.

Power: It took months to progress to doing dynamic exercises such as squats, any hanging exercises for abs, kettlebell squats, or swings and HIIT exercises.

If I pushed too hard too soon, I experienced pain and muscle spasm. I had to move slowly and overload gradually to build intensity over time. But the progression is simple and beneficial when followed:

Mobility → Stability → Functional Movement → Strength → Power

BOTTOM LINE

Increase your exercise levels with both cardiovascular and resistance training. To keep momentum, work around injuries, pain, or dislikes in a way that does not cause additional injury. Don't focus on what you don't like or can't do. Focus on what you do like and can do and watch the results that come when you steadily and slowly increase your levels of exercise.

BIG IDEAS

We are made to move, and movement is needed to heal or stay healthy.

We must work within limitations and around injuries.

Extreme pain, especially in tendons and/or joints, is a sign your intensity is too high or of bad technique or injury.

ACTION STEPS

Stay active. Keep going to the gym with minor injuries as you are able. Plan your workout around what you can do.

Target injured areas and use the gym and health care professionals (physical therapists, chiropractors, etc.) to rehab.

Constantly evaluate and adjust your workouts in a way that increases intensity over time but avoids and overcomes injuries.

SPRINT TO WIN

The Last Sprint: January I–February 20, 2020

*A goal is a dream with a finish line. –*DUKE ELLINGTON [61]

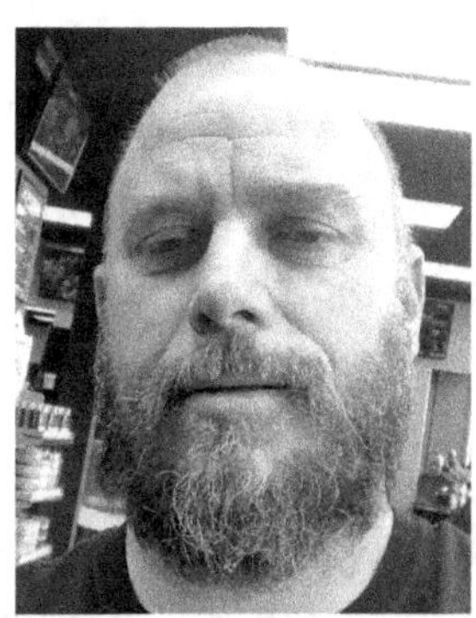 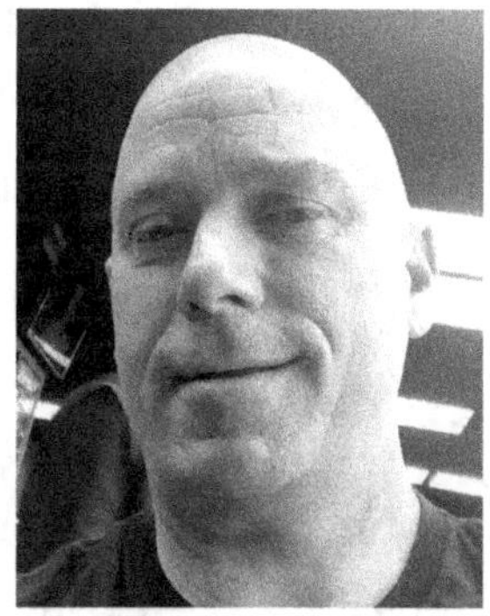

On December 26, 2019, I went to my barber, Nick, and asked him to shave my head and my beard. Some people literally didn't recognize me. I put myself in boot camp just as 2020 rolled in: a new decade. I was turning fifty on February 20, and it was game on. I started the journey back in 2018 and progressed along the way, but now it was time to go all in.

With several injuries and other setbacks, I had gone from 228 to a low of 210 on December 24, 2019. In that time, I had been consistent with going to the gym and using the elliptical three to four days a week. My August injury (sprained spine) had improved enough to do light weight machines and elliptical but not a whole lot more. Anything strenuous (kettlebell or dynamic lifting or HIIT) wasn't possible. I had to do boot camp with limitations.

By January 1, 2020, I was up to 214 from the holidays, so I had twenty-four pounds to lose in about seven weeks. I knew the first five pounds was holiday weight that would drop off easily, but I would still have about nineteen pounds to burn off. Even so, I was ready.

PROGRESSIVE OVERLOAD FOR GREATER RESULTS

A winning mindset is determined to find a way; I had to change up what I was doing if I wanted my results to change and accelerate. Instead of lifting whole body Monday, Wednesday, and Friday, I started splitting up muscle groups to do chest, legs, and abs on Monday, Wednesday, and Friday, and back, shoulders, and arms on Tuesday, Thursday, and Saturday. This shocked my body to build more muscle by adding both frequency and intensity to my resistance training. I also increased the frequency and/or intensity of my cardio to burn more fat. This was done by increasing time on the elliptical. I also got more intentional about healthier snacks with my bag of "rabbit food" traveling with me almost daily. If you want to break a plateau, you have to find a fresh approach.

To make further progress, consider how to get to the next level. Look again at food choices and exercise levels. What can you increase or rework? I would like to say I lost thirty-eight pounds in thirty-eight weeks, but that's not what happened. It was like 228 to 210 was a season and then I bounced back and forth between 210 and 215. Then I had to double down on my efforts and increase consistency to break 210.

Along the way, I had multiple injuries and life demands that sidetracked me. This led to bad weeks and literally bad months in terms of food choice and exercising. I had to keep from becoming discouraged or even quitting.

190 BY 2/20/20

To drop this weight, I needed to change my game plan and get focused for the next seven weeks. Never before had I set a target in terms of weight loss within a certain time frame, so this was brand new to me. I was confident that I had built a good cardiovascular base, and my muscles and joints, besides my back, were all in good condition for more strenuous activity and some significant dietary changes. Previous activity level and eating changes had built a base to prepare me for new and more strenuous habits and weight-loss techniques.

AT LEAST THIRTY MINUTES OF CARDIO
FOR FIFTY-ONE DAYS

I committed to doing the elliptical at least thirty minutes a day from January 1 to February 20. You should have seen the faces and heard the reactions when I shared this goal. From doubt to rebuke, people asked why, advised against it, and recommended other types of training, but I was all in. My reasoning was simple: it's math. You burn calories and fat doing cardiovascular training. You can't wish or pray fat away; it needs to be physically broken down, and cardio does that. It also put me in a constant fat-burning mode. It started with thirty minutes, and about ten to eleven days into it, I felt a shift in energy, outlook, and ability. After about two weeks, I increased to thirty-five minutes a couple of days a week, then forty. Then for the last three to four weeks, I bumped it up to sixty minutes every day unless I was excessively tired or had a time constraint. I was on that elliptical on my days off from work, before work, and even on my lunch break. The commitment was huge but gave me great momentum.

DIETARY CHANGES

I am not a diet guy in the sense of restricting food or using decreased eating as the main driver of weight loss, but in boot camp, I made some major dietary shifts along with greatly increased exercise levels.

DANIEL FAST

One of the things we do at my church is start the new year with a Daniel Fast to get spiritually focused. There are bonus health benefits from eating a plant-based diet for twenty-one days. My three-week Daniel Fast went from January 3-23, and I dropped six pounds (from 211 to 205). This was a disappointment because in years past, I dropped ten to twelve pounds without doing all the cardio I was currently doing. I learned my body had changed with age and in how it processed carbohydrates. I modified my eating within the Daniel Fast to lose weight by decreasing or cutting out dried fruit, like apricots, craisins, and raisins, and limiting nuts, like walnuts, cashews, and almonds. In years past, I could eat all I wanted of these and still drop weight. Though it was less weight than I expected, it was still a solid six-pound loss.

WEIGHT TRAINING SIX DAYS A WEEK

One of the dangers of cutting weight is possibly cutting muscle. If you diet alone without resistance training, you will cut a large amount of muscle, which is disastrous in the long run. A great metabolism is built and maintained with max muscle and low fat storage. I spent about fifteen to twenty minutes Monday through Saturday doing weight machines and free weights. My goal was not to build a large amount of muscle but to maintain what I had. One of the reasons I may have only lost six pounds during my Daniel Fast could have been that I was building muscle. This is the time period when people commented on my weight loss. So, a small weight loss combined with some new muscle may not get results on the scale, but it gets results health wise and in how you look. Overall, the Daniel Fast, increased weight training, and increased cardio put me in a great place for the final push.

MY COACHES

I needed additional coaching if I was going to make my goal. My methods up to this point were effective but too slow to reach my goal in my desired time frame. I was also willing to do some short-term, higher-stress dieting and exercise programs to reach my goals. Since I was in new territory, I sought out two friends who are also personal trainers: Bristol Jenkins and EJ Frain. I asked them both the same questions, got their advice, and then applied it to my situation and circumstances. Remember, losing weight is math and science but it is also an art; you must find what works for each individual.

They both recommended doing limited- or zero-carb days and also intermittent fasting. Both of these suggestions have recently become popular and mainstream. Honestly, I was skeptical to some degree but willing to try because I hoped to lose the last fifteen pounds at a fast pace. We isolated three main factors that could get me closer to my goal quickly:

1. Sixty minutes of daily cardio
2. Low- and no-carb days (carb cycling)
3. Intermittent fasting

LOW- AND NO-CARB DAYS

Honestly, this was 100 percent new to me in practice. Yes, I normally limit carbs, especially simple carbs, but have never had a no-carb day. In fact, I was somewhat opposed to the concept as unsustainable. To my surprise, it was extremely effective in helping me lose the last fifteen pounds in a short time span. I still wouldn't recommend it as a starting point, especially if you are not in good condition, but it worked extremely well for me on a short-term basis.

Three days a week (Monday, Wednesday, and Friday), I either totally eliminated or had miniscule carbs. The other days of the week, I kept my meals pretty much no carb but ate fruits and drank vegetable juice. To my surprise, I had high energy. From February 2-9, I went from 205 to 197, and then from February 9-16, my weight fell from 197 to 193. Then I did Monday, Tuesday, and Wednesday no carb and went from 193 on February 16 to 188 on February 20.

INTERMITTENT FASTING

I had lost six pounds on the Daniel Fast (vegetable-based diet) in three weeks. In the grand scheme of things, this is a healthy amount of weight to lose in this time period. I felt good, was eating well, and had made great physical progress doing cardio every day and lifting five to six days a week. I believe this set me up for the final four-week sprint to my goal.

Intermittent fasting simply means choosing to eat within an eight-hour time frame and fasting the other sixteen hours of the day. I chose to eat between noon and eight o'clock at night. My reasoning was that I needed to be able to work hard in the afternoon and then be strong and in a good mood until ten or eleven at night while with my family or working. It was practical because I could go to noon with good energy and then eat three to four times within this window.

To my happy surprise, I quickly learned it was not only practical but also highly effective. On the practical side, I was almost never hungry. I could go to noon without eating and be fine. Then I would eat three to four protein-based meals before eight o'clock. On Tuesday, Thursday, Saturday, and Sunday, I'd also have fruit and vegetable juice in between meals.

I have been fasting periodically for the past twenty years at our church for spiritual reasons. I think this helped me have success with intermittent fasting as I had conditioned my body to fast. One of the types of fasts we often do at church is a one-meal-a-day fast. I would choose dinner, meaning I would pray during normal breakfast and lunch times and then eat dinner. I never knew this discipline would later help me in my weight-loss goals.

THE FINAL WEIGH-IN

When I set the February 20 date for my goal weight, most people thought it was unrealistic; honestly, I had some doubts myself. I was committed to the weight and goal date, but I didn't know how I was going to get there. I started this process at forty-eight years old, and my plan was to lose one pound a week for thirty-five weeks. The original title for this book was *Losing Thirty-Five at Forty-Eight*; then age forty-nine came, and as I closed in on fifty, the title became *50 & Fit*.

In the big picture, I lost the first twenty-three pounds through simple changes in diet and exercise over time. Increased cardio and ongoing resistance training greatly decreased body fat and added muscle. I don't have body composition testing, but if I added seven pounds of muscle in the past year or so from resistance training, that would mean seven pounds of new muscle and thirty pounds less fat. Overall, that's huge physical progress.

SEVENTEEN POUNDS IN FOUR WEEKS

Basically, I lost twenty-three pounds the old-fashioned way with better eating and more exercise. Then I lost the last seventeen pounds in four weeks with intermittent fasting and full keto three days a week and modified keto the other four days, adding whole fruits and vegetables and some vegetable juice. By this time, I had been training my body to burn fat and was now ready to go full speed to the finish line. Below is my recorded weight from 2017-2018 and then from 10/30/19–2/20/20.

190 BY FEBRUARY 20, 2020

2018 bodyweight demonstrates minor changes. I was in a cycle of losing a little, then gaining a little more back:

12/30/17:   219
1/2/18:   220
1/3/18:   219
1/8/18:   218
1/29/18:   214
2/12/18:   213
2/14/18:   214
2/16/18:   214
11/14/18:   226
11/19/18:   225   *(This is when I committed to losing thirty-five pounds to get to 190.)*

2019-2020 Bodyweight:
10/30/19:   219
12/24/19:   210
12/31/19:   212
1/1/20:   214
1/2/20:   212
1/3/20:   211   *(Start of three-week Daniel Fast)*

1/5/20:   212
1/7/20:   210
1/8/20:   210
1/9/20:   210
1/12/20:   210
1/14/20:   210
1/16/20:   209
1/17/20:   210
1/20/20:   210
1/21/20:   209
1/22/20:   209
1/23/20:   208
1/25/20:   205   *(Last day of Daniel Fast [start 211 to finish 205])*
1/26/20:   207
1/28/20:   204
2/1/20:   207   *(After Phoenix trip)*
2/2/20:   205
2/4/20:   203
2/6/20:   201
2/7/20:   200
2/8/20:   199
2/9/20:   197
2/11/20:   198
2/13/20:   194
2/14/20:   194
2/15/20:   192
2/16/20:   193
2/17/20:   193
2/18/20:   192

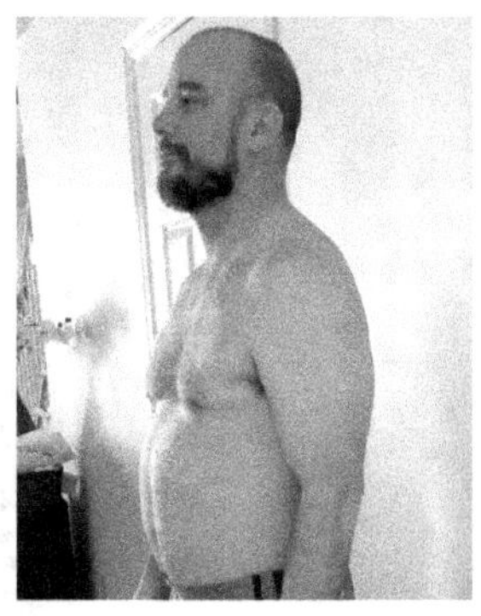

BEFORE

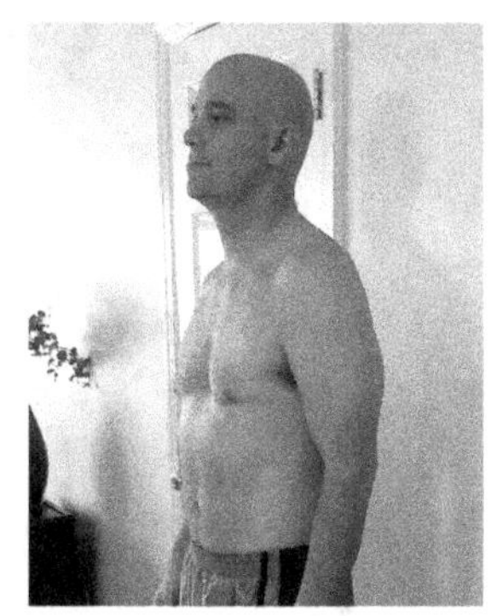

AFTER

2/19/20:   190
2/20/20:   188

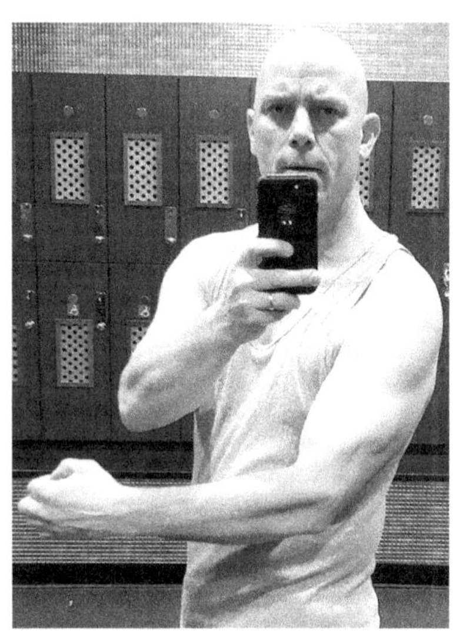

February 20, 2020 @ 188 pounds

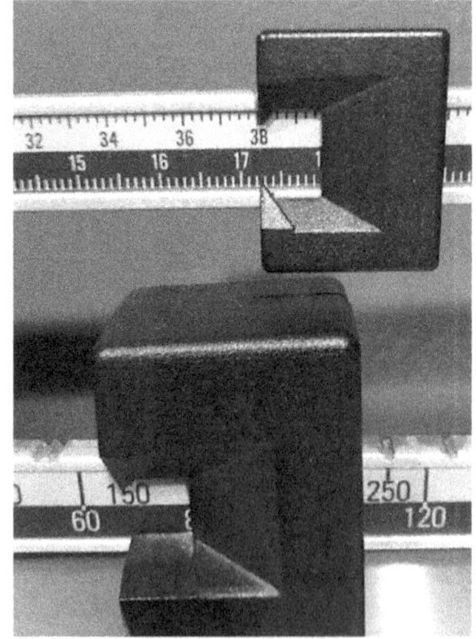

Bottom line: My vision and dream was to hit and maintain 190 pounds and to increase my daily energy levels. I dreamed, built the plan, and then executed the plan. From 228 to 188, I followed established physiological processes (science), put the work in and burned the fat (math), and made it work in my complicated and overly busy life (art). My success was guaranteed as I always returned to our three basic principles:

1.   **Build muscle:** our fat-burning engine
2.   **Burn fat:** through exercise and eating right
3.   **Eat right:** eating the right foods at the right times

Simple patterns over time get results. My hope is that you're dreaming of what a better life with less fat and more daily energy will look like. Make a plan and then execute that plan. You have the knowledge. You have the framework. Now it's time to get after it!

BIG IDEAS

Focused fat-burning sprints can help you make significant short-term progress.

Look for coaches in your process; this could include videos, articles, or people you know.

Formulate a plan to reach your next short- or long-term goal.

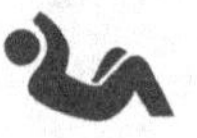

ACTION STEPS

Work your plan. Consistency over time is needed.

Modify your plan if it is not working.

Go all in to reach your goal.

WIN THE LONG WAR

Losing weight is hard. Maintaining weight is hard.
Staying overweight is hard. Choose your hard. [62]

When I set out to reach 190 pounds, I didn't view this as an event but as a new normal and lifestyle that would last for decades. In warfare, the terms *short war* and *long war* are used. More frequently, we use the saying, "You can win the battle but lose the war." The idea of winning the long war means planning and doing what it takes to win in the end. My long war means having a high energy level and healthy bodyweight for the next four to five decades. I'm not merely trying to be cute or muscular for summer. Up and down yo-yo dieting is winning the battle but losing the war.

PAIN OF DISCIPLINE OR REGRET?

We either choose the pain of discipline now or the pain of regret later. If you ignore the pain of discipline, it decreases, goes away, and gets replaced by the joy of discipline and the rewards it brings. Choosing the short-term pain of discipline always hurts less and gets better results than the long-term, lasting pain of regret.

REESTABLISHING MY BODYWEIGHT SET POINT

After hitting my goal of 190 in February, I had two goals for the month of March: reset and maintain my bodyweight at 190; get my back to 100 percent. My goal was not to *reach* 190; rather, my goal was to *stay* at 190. Substitute your own goal number; it may be less or more. You do you. You be the best you and do what you need to be healthy and happy.

Before and during March, the comments I heard most were not to lose too much and to stop losing. Others told me to keep losing, or when I was sitting, they'd point to my belly and comment that it looked like I "still had" a belly or my belly "was coming back."

MY GOAL HELPED ME STAY FOCUSED

Remember, my goal for the month of March was to stay at 190—not lose or gain. My goal was to reset my bodyweight at 190 so I could stay at 190 for years to come.

My other goal was to rehab my back. I had sprained my spine, which put me out of commission for about two months and severely limited what I could do for over six months. One of the reasons I lived on the elliptical was because that was what I could do. Dynamic or intense exercise put me into two to three days of pain. I now had to learn additional core strengthening exercising and programs for my abdominals and back.

Because my goal was clear, my mind was clear. I didn't listen to the voices of others or even my own feelings. One ninety with a healthy back was my goal. Learning, growing, and getting better is part of the game if you want to live differently. I had to be diligent in doing things I didn't feel like doing, but when you have a clear, committed goal, you do what you have to do to get there.

WHAT IS YOUR SET POINT?

Set point is the metabolic rate and bodyweight your body thinks are normal; therefore, your body tries to maintain this set point as your body is designed to survive. Your body doesn't have an opinion about how you look; it just wants to survive and be healthy. It is designed to seek a stable, normal state. The great news is, we can reset our normal metabolic rate and bodyweight.

WHY PEOPLE YO-YO DIET

Many people lose a good amount of weight only to gain it back and then some because the loss was accomplished through excessive calorie and nutrition restriction. Restrictive diets work at first because of math: eat fewer calories than you burn, and you will lose weight. But there are two basic problems with this approach:

1. Your body sees this restriction as starvation and slows down your metabolism (the rate at which you burn calories) while also breaking down your healthy muscle tissue for energy (gluconeogenesis); both are bad for you in the long term.

2. Your set point never changed, so if you dropped from two hundred fifty to two hundred, your body thinks your normal is two hundred fifty, so when you start eating normally again, your body is on a mission to get back to its normal weight: two hundred fifty. On top of that, your body often overcompensates and packs on even more weight, so your set point is

changed to a heavier weight.

MY FIRST TWENTY-THREE WAS SLOW AND STEADY

I spent over a year losing the first twenty-three pounds—a good approach because when you lose weight slowly and in a healthy manner, your set point is changed gradually, and your body makes healthy adjustments. Over that year, I added muscle, decreased bodyfat, and strengthened my heart, lungs, and muscles in a way that prepared me for my final sprint.

Remember that your weight on a scale and your body composition are two different things. I lost twenty-three pounds, but I was lifting weights, doing kettlebells, and other resistance exercises to gain muscle. Let's say that I put on ten pounds of muscle over the course of the year. That would mean my twenty-three-pound weight loss was a thirty-three-pound fat loss and a ten-pound muscle gain, which has huge health benefits and would result in a much healthier set point and overall body condition.

At this point, 205 was my new set point because it had been slow and steady. Let's say I overrestricted to get down to 190 and my body rebounded back to my set point. Because I had reestablished my set point at 205 instead of the 228 I started at, a rebound would be back to 205 instead of 228.

I NEVER SKIPPED MEALS

For the first twenty-three pounds, I never skipped a meal. I always ate breakfast, lunch, and dinner and usually ate several snacks. This provided my body with healthy nutrition and ensured progress was healthy and lasting. I had two goals in my food choices:

1. Reduce calories by decreasing fat, sugar, and processed foods.

2. Supply my body with sufficient nutrients to be healthy.

My main goal was to be healthy; the weight-loss part was just part of the process to reach greater health. Eating sufficient nutrients throughout the day not only supplies the body with what it needs to be strong and healthy, but it also minimizes times of hunger, which lead to snacking on junk food or overeating at mealtimes. This is extremely helpful emotionally as well. If you are not feeling hungry and deprived, you keep a more positive outlook and keep momentum going.

THE LAST SEVENTEEN POUNDS IN FOUR WEEKS

Yes, I lost seventeen pounds in four weeks, but I don't want people to think it was easy to lose or keep off. Here are a few things that made my forty-pound weight loss successful:

1. I lost twenty-three pounds slowly over the course of over a year through regular cardiovascular and resistance training, proper food choice, and gradual, ongoing increases in intensity level.

2. I consistently ate meals and snacks to provide nutrition and build and maintain a healthy metabolism.

3. I purposely burned fat—instead of just losing weight—positioning myself for extreme fat burning over the last month.

Following a keto diet Monday, Wednesday, and Friday, and adding fruits and vegetables on Tuesday, Thursday, Saturday, and Sunday, gave me adequate nutrition while I experienced tremendous fat burning.

FOOD TIMING, NOT SKIPPING MEALS

Eating only between noon and eight o'clock at night allowed me to burn fat sixteen hours a day and still eat three meals at noon, four, and eight, with vegetable and fruit snacks four days a week. This approach kept my metabolism flying without excessive muscle loss. Once again, I did not skip a meal. I restricted calories and made the right food choices, but every single day, I ate at least three times to provide my body with nutrients while still making my goal weight.

Then, when I decreased activity and ate a more regular diet, I was able to maintain the 190 pounds because the extreme fast loss of seventeen pounds in four weeks did not damage my metabolism and allowed me to return to a more normal exercise rate of four to five times per week and a more regular eating schedule—both time and food choice—and still maintain my goal weight.

SET POINT RE-ESTABLISHED

What this all tells us is that by returning to a more regular routine and maintaining my goal bodyweight, my body accepted and maintained 190 pounds as my new set point. If you ask me how I achieved success and maintenance while many others fail to do so, I would point to two main factors. First, I lost the first twenty-three pounds slowly and in a healthy manner. Second, I went hardcore for four weeks only and then returned to a more normal routine. Those four weeks got me great results, but it was a short enough span that it didn't shut down my metabolism or cause me to rebound and gain forty to fifty pounds back. In fact, I gained nothing back because I did the right things both over the long haul and in the short sprint of four weeks.

This is where science kicked in. Knowing how the body reacts to our food choices and exercise levels was key to both my period of long, slow weight loss and my four-week hardcore sprint. The math side of the equation was forty to sixty minutes on the elliptical daily. I knew if I went hard enough long enough, the fat would burn.

Spending the next month ensuring my set point was reestablished was key in my long-term success of establishing my new normal as 190 pounds.

Remember the steps for achieving your goals: dream, plan, and execute. It was simple—not easy but simple. My hope is that you, too, can follow this path and establish a new normal of greater daily energy and health at your desired weight.

BIG IDEAS

Your weight loss is not an event but a new and better lifestyle.

Even when restricting calories, you must purposely eat sufficient nutrients for health.

Food choice and timing greatly influence weight loss.

ACTION STEPS

Focus on building a stronger, healthier body over time:
build muscle, burn fat, eat right, repeat.

Schedule and eat meals and snacks that give you
needed nutrition.

Put in the work to burn the fat:
planned, purposeful, and effective work.

ENDNOTES

CHAPTER 1

1   **Ernest Hemingway,** *The Old Man and the Sea.*

CHAPTER 2

2   https://www.fearlessmotivation.com/2016/07/05/12-powerful-growth-mindset-quotes-empower/

3   https://www.dictionary.com/browse/mindset?s=t

4   https://www.awakenthegreatnesswithin.com/35-inspirational-quotes-on-priorities/

CHAPTER 3

5   https://quoteinvestigator.com/2017/03/13/winning/

6   https://www.someecards.com/usercards/viewcard/i-dont-diet-and-exercise-i-eat-and-train-83aad/?tagSlug=sports

7   https://www.dictionary.com/browse/execute?s=t

8   https://www.womansday.com/health-fitness/womens-health/g3209/best-weight-loss-motivation/?slide=2

CHAPTER 4

9   https://www.britannica.com/science/calorie

10   https://www.mayoclinic.org/healthy-lifestyle/weight-loss/in-depth/calories/art-20048065

11   https://www.psychologytoday.com/us/blog/the-athletes-way/201506/hippocrates-was-right-walking-is-the-best-medicine

12   http://dl.clackamas.edu/ch106-06/metaboli.htm

CHAPTER 5

13   https://www.brainyquote.com/quotes/daniel_cormier_812707

14   https://www.dictionary.com/browse/perseverance?s=t

CHAPTER 6

15   https://www.goodreads.com/quotes/tag/normal

CHAPTER 7

16   https://www.brainyquote.com/quotes/leo_tolstoy_138476

17   https://www.dictionary.com/browse/homeostasis?s=t

CHAPTER 8

18   https://www.dictionary.com/browse/metabolism?s=ts

19   https://academic.oup.com/ajcn/article/81/1/3/4607611

20   https://www.unm.edu/~lkravitz/Article percent20folder/epocarticle.html

CHAPTER 9

21   https://www.azquotes.com/author/28368-Evelyn_Ashford

22   https://medical-dictionary.thefreedictionary.com/overload+principle

23   https://medical-dictionary.thefreedictionary.com/hypertrophy

24   https://www.dictionary.com/browse/atrophy

CHAPTER 10

25   https://www.fearlessmotivation.com/2018/07/24/darren-hardy-quotes/

26   https://www.ncbi.nlm.nih.gov/pubmed/25162652

27   https://www.ncbi.nlm.nih.gov/pubmed/27747847

28   https://www.ncbi.nlm.nih.gov/pubmed/24773393

29   https://www.ncbi.nlm.nih.gov/pubmed/24773393

30   https://www.dictionary.com/browse/gluconeogenesis?s=t

CHAPTER 11

31   https://www.wildsayings.com/healthy-eating-quotes/

32   https://www.mayoclinic.org/healthy-lifestyle/nutrition-and-healthy-eating/
in-depth/fiber/art-20043983

33   https://www.azquotes.com/quote/341339

34   https://www.webmd.com/diet/features/water-for-weight-loss-diet#1

CHAPTER 12

35   https://www.elitedaily.com/wellness/quotes-motivation-fitness-bikini-season/1425966

36   https://www.goodreads.com/author/quotes/10803973.Jocko_Willink

CHAPTER 13

37   https://www.brainyquote.com/quotes/robert_collier_108959

38   https://www.goodreads.com/quotes/7131790-a-year-from-now-you-will-wish-you-had-started

39   https://www.healthline.com/health/exercise-fitness/ideal-body-fat-percentage#for-men

40   https://www.webmd.com/diet/body-bmi-calculator

41   https://www.everydayhealth.com/news/10-amazing-facts-about-your-blood-vessels/

42   https://www.livestrong.com/article/312522-how-many-calories-are-in-a-big-mac-meal/

43   https://www.calorieking.com/us/en/foods/f/calories-in-sandwiches-burgers-turkey-sandwich-on-
whole-grain-bread/437PppHCTiCVTjaynCf4NQ

CHAPTER 15

44   https://www.physicsclassroom.com/class/newtlaws/Lesson-1/Newton-s-First-Law

CHAPTER 16

45   https://www.brainyquote.com/quotes/chuck_norris_773610?src=t_aging

46   https://www.mayoclinic.org/healthy-lifestyle/womens-health/in-depth/menopause-weight-
gain/art-20046058

47   https://quotefancy.com/quote/1283871/Jack-LaLanne-People-don-t-die-of-old-age-they-die-of-neglect

48   https://www.coolfunnyquotes.com/author/anonymous/didnt-mean-to-gain-weight/

CHAPTER 17

49   https://www.azquotes.com/quote/761094

50   https://everydaypower.com/sleep-quotes/

51   **N.F. Watson, M.S. Badr, G. Belenky**, et al., *"Recommended amount of sleep for a healthy adult: a joint consensus statement of the American Academy of Sleep Medicine and Sleep Research Society,"* Sleep (2015); 38(6):843–844.

CHAPTER 18

52   https://www.notsalmon.com/2015/11/30/stop-stress-eating/

CHAPTER 19

53   https://dustyholcomb.com/tag/carol-welch-baril/

54   https://motivationping.com/quote-dieting-weight-loss/

55   https://www.obesityaction.org/community/article-library/hypertension-and-obesity-how-weight-loss-affects-hypertension/

56   http://alkalinevalley.com/5-of-the-healthiest-alkaline-rolled-grains-you-can-eat-in-place-of-unhealthy-oatmeal/2/

57   https://www.ncbi.nlm.nih.gov/pubmed/382forty17

58   https://www.mayoclinic.org/diseases-conditions/depression/in-depth/depression-and-exercise/art-20046495

59   https://www.azquotes.com/quote/155028?ref=back-pain

60   http://www.proformathleticdevelopment.com/the-functional-movement-screen-injury-prevention-performance-enhancement/

CHAPTER 20

61   https://www.azquotes.com/quote/527791

CHAPTER 21

62   https://www.sparkpeople.com/resource/quotes_translation.asp?id=417

ENDNOTES

ABOUT THE AUTHOR

Jack Redmond is the Founder and President of **Redmond Strategy Group** which exists to help people: LIVE YOUR PURPOSE! Redmond Strategy Group accomplishes this through Life Coaching, organization consultation, leadership development and content creation.

He is an author, international speaker, Life Coach and trainer. He spent the past 25 years focused on fostering personal development, leadership and organizational growth.

Jack reached back to his former career and education in the area of health and fitness to produce *50 & Fit* with the goal of positioning individuals for greater health, increased daily energy along with a more enjoyable and productive life.

Jack, while based in the greater NY Metro region, travels throughout the United States and internationally to train leaders for greater community impact. Some of his greatest passions include mentoring young entrepreneurs and helping build stronger organizations through the following three step process:

Dream

You must see and define your vision.

Plan

Everything must be well thought out.

Execute

Your plan must be followed and adjusted as needed for success.

Part of peak performance occurs when an individual is at their personal best. Physical, emotional and mental health work together to maximize efficiency and productivity. By achieving greater personal health and increased daily energy, a person positions themselves for a better and more productive life.

For personal or corporate coaching or consultation, go to www.RedmondStrategyGroup.com